P9-ECW-057

About the Authors

Stacey J. Bell, D.Sc., R.D., is an Instructor in Surgery at Harvard Medical School, and Research Dietitian at Beth Israel Deaconess Hospital (a major teaching hospital for the Harvard Medical School), working primarily with patients with HIV infection and AIDS.

R. Armour Forse, M.D., Ph.D., is an Associate Professor of Surgery at Harvard Medical School; Chief, Division of Critical Care, Beth Israel Deaconess Hospital; Co-Director of the Harvard Center of Minimally Invasive Surgery; and Chief of the Surgical Metabolism Laboratory of Beth Israel Deaconess Hospital.

Each author has more than 20 years experience of counseling and treating patients for nutrition-related problems.

To Jay Blake, who inspired us to write this book.

Acknowledgments

We would like to acknowledge several people, for without their help it would not have been possible to write this book.

First, we would like to recognize the superb editing skills of Maria Sachs, who has been a scientific editor throughout her life. One of us (SJB) has been lucky enough to have her as a friend for many years. Maria spent hours editing the numerous drafts of the manuscript before it was even sent to the publisher. She has the wonderful ability to make even the most difficult, technical language easy to understand and flow. Maria is also a superb cook and spent considerable time working on Chapter 7, Meal Planning & Food Preparation. From sitting in on our nutritional counseling sessions with patients, Maria heard time and time that people want simple ways to put into practice what they learn. In these meal plans, Maria has captured what our patients have been asking for. We can't thank her enough.

Also, we would like to thank Estelle Raiffa, a friend of mine (SJB) for over 20 years. She has many fine qualities, but one of her best is her ability to cook—and can she cook! Fortunately for us, Estelle recently retired and volunteered to put together a few favorite recipes. This blossomed into more than a few, and soon Estelle was combing the greater Boston area and beyond for recipes suitable for people with HIV infection. We urge you to try the delectable meals in Chapter 8; each meets with our nutritious seal of approval.

Our luck continued when we hired a young dietitian, Jül Gerrior, who is also a well-trained athlete. Even better, we got two for the price of one—her twin sister is a certified exercise physiologist. Jül and Janel Gerrior have been instrumental in writing the exercise section in Chapter 2. You now have the latest thinking in how to exercise; and, perhaps more importantly, the information is appropriate for people with HIV infection no matter the stage of disease or current fitness level.

Finally, with any book there is a need to develop rapport with the publisher's editorial staff. Jon Ebersole and Jeff Braun have been exemplary. We have written several previous books and have never encountered two more talented writers and creative minds. These two have transformed an OK book into something that we believe reads better and certainly makes our message clearer. Special mention should be made of Jon, who totally immersed himself in this project. Every time we spoke, Jon prefaced his remarks with, "Last night I was thinking about *Positive Nutrition*, and I think we should...." He exceeded what any writer would expect from an editor.

Notice:
Consult your health care professional

Readers are advised to seek the guidance of a licensed physician or health care professional before making changes in health care regimens, since each individual case or need may vary. This book is intended for informational purposes only and is not for use as an alternative to appropriate medical care. While every effort has been made to ensure that the information is the most current available, new research findings, being released with increasing frequency, may invalidate some information.

Contents

introduction

If you learn just one thing from this book, make it this: With HIV infection, nutritional care is just as important as medical care. The two are intertwined, and if you ignore one, the other will suffer.

Scientists have made great strides in understanding the nutrition problems caused by HIV infection and AIDS. We know which treatments will overcome these problems. More importantly, you can take these steps to better nutritional care on your own, using the information here and working with your doctor. However, it is up to you to take charge. You've made the first step—you're reading this book; we know you are concerned about your health or the health of someone you care for. Now, you can do something about it.

Good nutrition—more specifically a positive, proactive nutritional approach for HIV infection and AIDS—is important because the infection itself disrupts your body's use of nutrients. Also, we know that some treatments of the infection actually impair nutritional health. The result? Your nutritional health deteriorates and your immune system declines, which leads to further problems.

But this doesn't have to happen. You can do a great deal to stay well nourished and active, in addition to being more resistant to further health problems. Furthermore, with the advent of new drug therapies, including antiretrovirals and protease inhibitors, more and more people can look forward to long, relatively symptom-free lives. These new therapies are most successful when sound nutritional health is maintained. This book shows you how.

The concept of Positive Nutrition is anchored in three principles that in many ways, go against conventional nutrition wisdom:

{principles of positive nutrition}

1. Decide each day how you are going to meet your macronutrient needs (protein, fat, carbohydrates) and spend less time on how you are going to meet your micronutrient needs (vitamins, minerals).

2. Ignore advertisements, bulletins, and articles aimed at the general public that trumpet information on healthy eating.

3. Follow a daily meal plan based on the Positive Nutrition Pyramid.

These principles, which will be explained thoroughly in this book, are based on scientific studies and designed specifically for people with HIV infection and AIDS.

This is probably your first exposure to this amount of sound nutrition advice. Perhaps you've been told or thought that feeling queasy or losing your appetite and weight were inevitable side effects of the infection and medications. Your doctor may have made a passing remark such as, "You look as if you've lost some weight, but that's part of the disease." Or perhaps you've heard, "All patients have a little diarrhea—that's just something you have to live with." This does not have to be the case.

Doctors who treat persons with HIV infection and AIDS are experts across all aspects of treatment, of which nutrition is just one. They are knowledgeable in medical-related issues such as antiretrovirals, antibiotics, and chemotherapy. They're also trained in diet-related problems—weight loss, diarrhea, and the like. However, sometimes the medical issues take precedence over the nutrition-related aspects of your health. This is wrong.

Tackling Nutrition Head-On

HIV infection produces malnutrition, which, if untreated, will cause your body to slowly starve itself. This malnutrition, however, is not a byproduct of HIV infection exclusively. It occurs in many other diseases, particularly cancer and severe infections.

Nearly 25 years ago—well before we were aware of AIDS—doctors and scientists started treating malnourished patients and researching the ideal diets to help them. Their extensive work with cancer and heart disease patients and accident and burn victims has taught us much. We've learned how to gauge the severity of malnutrition; we've learned about the macronutrient needs (protein and fat, for instance) and micronutrient needs (vitamins and minerals); and we've learned to provide specialized diets, including those that rely upon artificial foods. This knowledge has important implications for people with HIV infection and AIDS.

In short, malnutrition is treatable, as long as it is caught early—before you lose more than 20 percent of your usual weight. So don't wait for symptoms of malnutrition to occur. The ideal time to change your diet is when you learn that you are infected. However, you can benefit from this book no matter where you are in the disease.

We don't believe in holding back information, even if it is unpleasant. This book presents everything from the basic nutrients everyone with HIV infection needs to other forms of nutrition that may be needed in the later stages of AIDS, such as diets that are given by a feeding tube or through a vein. If you are newly diagnosed with no symptoms, for instance, you may not need or want to know what can be done if you're not feeling well. That's OK. There's plenty of information in the first few chapters, in particular, that will get you off to a good start in your nutritional care. However, we do think that knowing what may happen down the road will help you decide the best course to take today.

We have counseled hundreds of patients and learned a great deal about the nutrition problems, recurring complaints, and questions that people with HIV infection face. All of these are covered in this book. We tell you what works and what doesn't. In addition to outlining the Principles of Positive Nutrition, we provide sensible, easy meal planning tips that offer great variety. You'll also learn how to talk with your doctor about nutrition—a vital skill for take-charge people. Also, our patients have asked us to help them get through days when they don't feel well, so we include our advice here.

We designed *Positive Nutrition for* HIV *Infection and* AIDS as a reader-friendly, self-help guide that will enable you to take an active role in your own nutritional care. The information will also be useful for others in your life: family members, friends, your partner, community workers, outreach workers, volunteers who may provide meals at your home, and anyone else in your household. We think doctors, dietitians, nurses, social workers, and other health care professionals will also benefit from this book.

Our plan for Positive Nutrition has the greatest benefit for assertive people who stay aware of the latest treatments for HIV infection. If you are an active partner in your medical care now, becoming proactive in your nutritional care will be easy. If you're not there yet, this book will help you take a greater role in your nutritional care—which we hope will spill over into all aspects of your health care.

It is important to note that most of what we tell you about nutrition is not experimental. When information is speculative, we will let you know. But what you will learn here represents a combination of our experience and the results of studies published in scientific journals. Some of these articles were written by us, some by other professionals. In any case, before you make changes in your diet, talk with your doctor. And that applies not only to what we say in this book, but also to what others tell you.

Who Should You Turn To?

For nutrition information, the safest and soundest suggestions come from physicians and nurses who are specially trained in nutritional science and from dietitians. You'll undoubtedly get advice from other people who mean well, but their suggestions may not be for the best.

One man was told by friends that he should eat only brown rice and tea to "cleanse his body." At first he felt great, and his diarrhea disappeared. But when we saw him several months later, he had lost weight, felt fatigued, and was profoundly malnourished. We started extensive nutrition counseling and pointed out the pitfalls of eliminating major food groups like meat and dairy products. We then devised a special high-protein diet that did not irritate his gastrointestinal tract or make his diarrhea worse.

It took a few weeks before he trusted us enough to follow our instructions, but when he finally did, his weight and strength slowly increased. His friends had meant well, but their advice hurt him. Fortunately, in this case, the harm could be corrected.

By no means do we reject nontraditional therapies. However, we are leery of nontraditional therapies that have never been subjected to scientific testing for their use in HIV infection.

By no means do we reject nontraditional therapies. At the moment, for example, we are investigating the effect of ginseng and various oils such as fish and olive oil on infections. But since there are no conclusive answers yet on how these foods affect immunity, we discourage their use at present. We are leery of nontraditional therapies that have never been subjected to scientific testing for their use in HIV infection.

Making the Most of Positive Nutrition

We suggest that you use this book several ways. You may want to read it cover to cover, just to see what's in it. For specific questions about symptoms, you may choose to read a particular chapter. For instance, there may be days when you don't feel well because of a fever. After getting treatment from your doctor, you may find that the antibiotics cause diarrhea and you lose your appetite. At that point, it may be a good idea to review Chapter 5, When You Don't Feel Well.

The book also contains a chapter on meal planning and food preparation and another on recipes. We know that the best nutrition information in the world is useless if you can't put it into practice. For us, it comes down to this: Can you eat according to the guidelines we provide? We think so. The simple meals are designed to meet your special needs; for instance, the need for twice as much protein as you did before HIV infection.

To help you reach your nutritional goals, we give you lots of ideas on how to prepare a variety of foods quickly and easily—in less than 15 minutes. Our food preparation tips include a list of essential ingredients plus optional ingredients for each dish. By swapping these ingredients between dishes, you'll have dozens of ways of cooking a simple dish, say baked chicken. Furthermore, you probably already stock everything you'll need to prepare these dishes. If not, your local grocery store will have the necessary ingredients.

Finally, the last chapter features culturally diverse recipes. Each recipe was tested in a typical household kitchen for the serving size suggested. All are nutritionally sound and extremely tasty.

As you read on, consider yourself one of our patients under nutritional care here at Deaconess Hospital and Harvard Medical School. And remember, the more active you are in your own care, the more useful this program of Positive Nutrition will be.

adapting to your changing body

Why do you eat?

Don't worry, this isn't a trick question. If you said, "To live," you're on the mark.

To be more precise, though, nutrition is the process of consuming foods or food substitutes and of converting them into usable energy and proteins for the body to live.

With HIV infection, however, this process changes. Most often, the virus causes three nutritional problems: a diminished appetite, less efficient nutrient absorption, and changes in the way your body processes food. All of this can result in one thing—malnutrition.

In this chapter, we will help you understand your nutritional needs and how they are impacted by the progression of HIV infection. You will learn about malnutrition—how it develops and how to delay or limit it. We'll also discuss weight loss—one of the chief symptoms of malnutrition. Through it all, our goal is to lay the important groundwork for the Principles of Positive Nutrition, which we will formally introduce in Chapter 2.

How Malnutrition Develops

In its simplest sense, malnutrition means you are not getting proper nutrition; your body becomes malnourished.

Proper nutrition is needed because the body is continually repairing itself: making new blood, skin, and organ cells; storing calories as fat and then burning up the fat for energy; and creating byproducts such as urine and carbon dioxide. Every day there is new growth of hair, skin, and nails. Millions of new red and white blood cells are produced each hour, ready to transport oxygen or fight infections. Even the lining of the intestine is rapidly sloughing off old, used cells, allowing new ones to take their place. In fact, the entire intestinal surface is replaced with new cells every three to five days; this shows that the body goes to extremes to ensure that foods are adequately absorbed.

For all of these dynamic processes to occur at an optimal rate, the body needs to be supplied with a steady source of nutrients—but not just any nutrients. The body is particular about what it needs, at what times, and in what amounts. There is no "day off" from having to nourish your body.

HIV infection, however, changes the way your body works. For instance, as the virus spreads throughout the body, it makes the body more susceptible to other infections, known as secondary infections. Additionally, if you have HIV infection, you can become malnourished even if you eat the same foods in the same amounts as before your diagnosis.

Malnutrition is a very common problem for people with HIV infection. One of its most obvious symptoms is weight loss, which occurs in about 98 percent of all people with HIV infection. A little weight loss by itself is not so bad. But you must deal with it early because excessive weight loss does create problems. With a loss of over 20 percent of one's usual weight, the body is malnourished and can no longer work efficiently. Immunity declines and fatigue sets in. Once that happens, malnutrition is not easy to treat. So take charge and get help from your doctor as soon as possible; don't wait until you've dropped 20 pounds before you become concerned.

There are three reasons why people with HIV infection become malnourished:

+ *Loss of appetite*
+ *Inadequate absorption of nutrients by the intestine*
+ *Changes in how the body processes food*

We will discuss these changes in this chapter and ways to combat them in subsequent chapters.

Loss of Appetite

As we've mentioned, HIV infection causes people to lose their appetite, but there is more to it than simply not feeling hungry. The medical term for this condition is anorexia. Scientific evidence suggests that the virus itself causes a signal to be sent to the brain, saying, "don't eat." We suspect that substances known as cytokines cause this phenomenon, which also occurs with other infections and cancer.

The term "cytokines" is used to describe a group of many similar substances. You may have heard of the main ones that have been studied in HIV infection: interleukin-1 (IL-1), tumor necrosis factor (TNF), and interferon (INF).

When the body suffers an injury—whether a burn, infection, or surgical incision, or something minor like a bruise or irritated gums from tooth brushing—cytokines are released by the white blood cells, called monocytes. They are also released by various tissues that house cells called macrophages such as the liver, lung, and spleen. At the affected area, the cytokines stimulate the immune system and help cells work with each other to heal the "injury." This process takes place in everyone, practically all the time. The problem occurs when too many or too few cytokines are released.

Normally, a blood-brain barrier protects our brain cells from toxins and other substances that may adversely affect the brain. However, when there are too many cytokines in the system, which seems to happen with HIV infection, some cytokines are believed to penetrate this barrier. They affect the hypothalamus (the appetite center of the brain) in a way which causes a loss of appetite, producing anorexia. In addition, it appears that cytokines can actually speed up the progress of the HIV infection by causing the virus to replicate at a greater rate than normal.

In San Francisco, Drs. Mark Hellerstein and Carl Grunfeld have explored the relationship between cytokines and appetite. They found that rats injected with cytokines ate significantly less than normal. The animals reverted to eating a normal amount of food when treated with ibuprofen or a diet containing fish oil, or when the cytokine injections stopped. Interestingly, rats receiving cytokines for more than 7 days overcame the loss of appetite; they gradually regained their appetite over a few weeks until it was nearly normal. This shows that in animals, the body gets used to the presence of cytokines, and the effect on appetite diminishes with time.

Apparently the same thing happens in people with HIV infection. During HIV infection with no secondary infections, people adapt to the low level of cytokines and don't have anorexia. However, when a secondary infection occurs and a large number of cytokines are released, appetite decreases. After the secondary infection is treated, appetite usually returns to normal.

Cytokines affect not only the hypothalamus but also the stomach. When cytokines were injected into laboratory animals, the emptying ability of their stomachs decreased. This probably happens in people, too. Just think of the last time you had the flu or an infection—you may have felt "full" and not much like eating. The feeling of fullness contributes to the lack of appetite and weight loss.

Because loss of appetite and cytokine release are so strongly related, it is tempting to assume that the weight loss associated with HIV infection is also related to cytokines. However, that relationship is a little tenuous in humans. Some studies reported that there were higher amounts of blood cytokines during HIV infection than AIDS, while other studies found the opposite. Stepped-up cytokine activity does, however, seem to cause muscle wasting (see Protein and Wasting, page 11).

The conflicting reports about cytokine levels in people with HIV infection may be explained by the fact that is very difficult to accurately measure these substances. Most cytokines stay in the blood for only about 15 minutes. Then, they are picked up by something called a receptor; when that happens, the cytokine becomes undetectable. The number of cytokines released from macrophages indicates overall cytokine activity better than cytokines floating in the blood, but these tissue measurements are obtainable only from laboratory animals after the animal is sacrificed. In people, the best we can do is to isolate the white blood cells from other blood cells and measure how many cytokines they release.

Still, numerous investigators, including us, are working to develop a clearer understanding of the relationship between cytokines, HIV infection, and anorexia. And efforts are being made to counterbalance the action of the cytokines so as to improve appetite and to slow the disease process.

In the meantime, understanding the process will help you choose appropriate treatments. If anorexia is the sole reason for weight loss, appetite stimulants will usually be prescribed. After 2 months of treatment, you and your doctor should evaluate the effectiveness of the therapy.

There are two approved drugs for stimulating appetite in HIV infection: Marinol (Roxane Labs, Columbus OH) and Megace (Bristol Myers Squibb, Princeton, NJ). Both are effective but each has side effects, which affect patients differently. Thus, if the first choice is unsuccessful at the 2-month evaluation, the second may be prescribed.

Marinol is a synthetic version of the active ingredient found in marijuana. The manufacturer claims that the drug stimulates appetite, not weight gain; it induces the "munchies." This drug is legal and is not habit forming in the doses that stimulate appetite. The catch is that you may need to wait 2 weeks until it works. It may also treat nausea that may occur from some of the medications you are taking.

> *If anorexia is the sole reason for weight loss, appetite stimulants will usually be prescribed.*

Some patients get a little "high" from the Marinol, but not enough to impair their thinking at work or their driving ability. To those of our patients who are reluctant to take it, we often suggest taking half the dose (one 2.5 mg pill) before they go to bed. This leaves their days clear of the drug and helps them to sleep. Once people adjust to this dose, they take a 2.5 mg pill every 12 hours.

The other appetite stimulant, Megace, was found to stimulate appetite, quite by accident, in a study in which women with breast cancer were given it for other reasons. All the women complained that they gained weight from the drug. Two large-scale studies in people with HIV infection show that Megace causes weight gain. However, that weight is mostly fat, not muscle, so it will not make you stronger. Large doses (400 - 800 mg) of Megace are required, so it costs slightly more than Marinol.

There is a current study in which patients are taking Marinol and Megace together. The hope is that the best effect of both drugs will be obtained: appetite increase and weight gain. Since both drugs have few side effects, you should ask your physician about taking one or both when you have lost 5 pounds as a result of no appetite. Most of our patients keep a supply of each on hand and take them as needed when they aren't hungry.

Malabsorption and Diarrhea

The problem of malabsorption is the second reason why people with HIV infection become malnourished. Malabsorption, as its name suggests, occurs when nutrients are not absorbed normally. To understand why this happens, and how it can lead to malnutrition, a quick lesson is needed regarding the digestion process.

The body's digestive system is a complex and well-controlled system that breaks food down into a form the body can use: most carbohydrates are broken down into glucose; protein into amino acids; and fats (triglycerides) into fatty acids. This digestive process begins in your mouth and continues as food particles pass from the stomach to the small intestine. (The colon—also known as the large intestine—is next in line, but only minimal digestion takes place there.)

After being broken down, nutrients are absorbed into the bloodstream for energy. Most nutrients are normally absorbed through the walls of the small intestine. The few that remain, such as fiber and water—along with intestinal digestive juices—move to the colon. Here, some salts, vitamins, and water are absorbed. Undigested food, water, and dead bacteria (which are naturally present), form into stool.

This process of digestion is how your body gets energy and maintains life. With HIV infection, however, the small intestine or colon may be damaged by parasites, bacteria, funguses, or viruses, including the HIV infection itself.

If the colon is damaged, it cannot absorb water, sodium, and other minerals as it normally should.

If the small intestine is damaged, your body misses out on properly absorbing fat and the nutrients that normally would be absorbed with fat—for example, fat-soluble vitamins such as beta-carotene and vitamin A. The absorption of complex carbohydrates, such as those found in bread, pasta, pastries, and potatoes, is also disrupted.

In addition, some protein is lost when the small intestine is damaged, but only when the damage is severe. The body makes every attempt to nourish itself, even in the face of disease. Because protein is vital for maintaining the body cells and functions, the small intestine's highest priority is to absorb protein at all costs, even at the expense of malabsorbing other, less important nutrients like fat and carbohydrates. (You'll learn more about the importance of protein in Chapter 2.)

One of the major dietary advances in treating malabsorption problems of the small intestine is the discovery of an easily digestible fat called a medium-chain triglyceride (MCT). Fat is the most difficult nutrient to digest, and a pathogen in the small intestine almost always leads to some fat-absorption problems. But MCT fats are not difficult to absorb; they are chemically different and do not require sophisticated digestion.

The medium in medium-chain triglyceride refers to the number of carbon atoms on a fatty acid of the triglyceride. Conventional fats usually contain 16 carbons or more and are called long-chain triglycerides. The longer the chain of carbons, the more difficult the fat is to digest. MCT fats, with only 8 to 12 carbons, are easy to digest and safe. They are even put into many baby formulas.

Dr. Christine Wanke at Deaconess Hospital in Boston, has studied the use of an MCT-rich formula called Lipisorb in fighting malabsorption caused by AIDS. She found that the MCT fats in this nutritional supplement (made by Mead Johnson) were much better absorbed than conventional fats. Patients were given Lipisorb for

12 days; their absorption of fat calories improved so much that it seems likely it will produce weight gain if used for the long term. We will talk in more detail about this and other oral supplements containing MCT fats in Chapter 6.

Fat absorption problems should be addressed in your diet. However, even during times of severe fat malabsorption we lose in bowel movements no more than 10 percent of the fat we consume. This means that if your daily diet contains 50 grams of fat (the Positive Nutrition plan recommends getting *at least* 50 grams each day), the most you could lose is 5 grams of fat, which is equal to only 45 calories.

Besides absorption problems and the loss of nutrients, a damaged digestive system will likely cause one of two types of diarrhea: small bowel diarrhea or colonic diarrhea.

Small bowel diarrhea occurs when the small intestine is damaged by a pathogen or "bug." The presence of a pathogen will also cause an overabundance of digestive juices to be released. These overwhelm the colon, further exacerbating diarrhea.

As you may recall, the small intestine allows food particles to be digested and nutrients absorbed. When it is damaged, both of these processes are hampered. Food that normally would be digested and absorbed moves to the colon. There, nonharmful bacteria that are naturally present begin to digest what food particles they can, but because the colon is not designed to digest great amounts of food, problems occur. A lot of air is produced, which you may feel as bloating. The effect: Water and any excess food that is not digested by the colonic bacteria leaves as a diarrheal bowel movement.

With colonic diarrhea, the small intestine works fine—digesting and absorbing nutrients properly. Pathogens in the colon, however, irritate the colon and interfere with the its main job, the absorption of water. The effect: watery diarrhea.

You and your doctor's approach to treating the absorption problems and diarrhea depends on which part of the intestine is damaged. If it's the colon only, you may lose water and some salts, become dehydrated, and feel weak. Water loss can quickly cause weight loss. However, once you take in fluids to replace these losses, your weight will go up. A damaged small intestine is more serious because it is responsible for digesting and absorbing most of the nutrients you consume.

For many people, weight loss and malnutrition come from the lack of appetite associated with malabsorption and its resulting diarrhea. Although it's natural to not want to eat in order to avoid having an accident, appetite stimulants are not the answer. In fact, they should not be used until further evaluations are made and the diarrhea is corrected.

It takes a long time, sometimes years, for malabsorption to lead to anorexia and finally malnutrition. Fortunately, before that, malabsorption can be treated. The key is knowing what's causing the problem: the small intestine, colon, or both.

The first step may be to have your stool analyzed for pathogens, which can be treated with antibiotics. Another test is a fecal fat test, which helps diagnose fat absorption problems. A d-xylose test will reveal any carbohydrate-absorbing problems. In addition, a gastroenterologist can take a visual biopsy of the small intestine and determine if a pathogen is affecting it.

Sometimes the symptoms of small bowel diarrhea will disappear in response to direct treatment of an organism, say a parasite. Other times, the diarrhea will have no known origin, making it "path-negative" diarrhea. In this case, you may receive an antidiarrheal medication and be asked to try to control it through diet.

As we said, it can take years before the malabsorption of foods leads to anorexia and malnutrition. Still, malabsorption can and should be treated. In Chapter 5, we'll give you guidelines on how to eat when you have diarrhea, and in Chapter 6, we'll suggest oral supplements to use during those times.

Changes in How the Body Processes Foods

The third way HIV infection causes malnutrition is the most intrusive: it disrupts the overall function of the body. The virus changes the body's metabolism—how it processes foods.

As we have explained, the virus somehow causes the body to waste some of the foods you eat, especially fat. When this happens, the food that would usually go into nourishing your cells takes a different, unproductive pathway. Left uncorrected, the body starves itself. But this starvation differs from other types of starvation; for instance, the kind seen in protesters who fast. If you fast when you are well, you generally lose 80 percent fat and 20 percent protein from muscle. If starvation accompanies disease, though, the weight loss is split about evenly between fat and muscle.

Why the difference? Again, cytokines appear to be the culprits. We know that cytokines are released in the presence of infection or injury and can lead to a depressed appetite and anorexia. But they do more than that; cytokines also disrupt metabolism. Unfortunately, very little is known why this happens or how to correct it. Nonetheless, faulty processing of food is the greatest contributor to malnutrition—even more than anorexia and malabsorption. And it usually strikes three areas: fat metabolism, protein metabolism, and calorie needs.

FATS—Most of the fats in your diet are triglycerides. Normally they are broken down by the small intestine and transported to tissues, including the liver, for energy or stored for later use. At the same time, the liver produces small amounts of fats and releases them to the bloodstream. HIV infection upsets this process, however, causing the liver to put too many fats into your bloodstream. The fats literally circulate round and round, day after day, without being captured for energy or storage.

> *There is really nothing wrong with high triglycerides levels if you aren't losing weight. Unfortunately, if weight loss occurs, there is yet no treatment to correct the defects in fat metabolism.*

Triglycerides are usually cleared from the blood and carried to storage by specific proteins called lipoprotein lipases. Extensive animal studies at Dr. Carl Grunfeld's lab in San Francisco suggest that when disease is present, these protein carriers are defective or the body makes too few. Another explanation may be that because the liver goes haywire and uncontrollably produces a lot of triglycerides—lipoprotein lipase production simply cannot keep up. Some of the triglycerides may go into storage only to be quickly shuttled back out again to the blood. This shuttling of fats consumes calories and may exacerbate weight loss. And all of this—the high triglycerides in the blood and low level of lipoprotein lipases—is caused by cytokines.

In Chapter 4, Tests and Measurements—Working with Your Doctor, we recommend that you have the triglyceride levels in your blood tested every 6 months. If they are elevated, you may have faulty fat metabolism. Many of our patients do. It is nothing to worry about and is not usually treated; it simply confirms that the virus changes how your body uses fat. The same high triglyceride levels are also seen in people who have been severely injured in an accident or those who have undergone extensive surgery. There is really nothing wrong with high triglyceride levels if you aren't losing weight. Unfortunately, if weight loss occurs, there is yet no treatment to correct fat metabolism defects, but work is going on this area.

PROTEIN AND WASTING—Another disturbance in how the body processes foods has to do with proteins. As you know, proteins from food are usually absorbed quite easily. The trouble occurs afterward, when the proteins stored in the muscles are immediately drawn out again. Once more, cytokines are to blame for this action, which was identified first at Deaconess Hospital by Drs. Nawfal Istfan and Bruce Bistrian. Although the proteins are eventually excreted in the urine, the entire process consumes calories and leads to muscle wasting. In fact, weight loss during HIV infection is due partly to protein lost through stepped-up cytokine activity.

The sole reason we eat protein is to make new tissues in the body. Every day, the body manufactures new proteins and gets rid of used-up proteins. This process is quite efficient; for every gram of protein that is broken down (catabolized), a gram of protein is made (synthesized). So, the ratio of protein synthesis to protein catabolism should be 1 to 1. During infections such as HIV infection or cancer, however, increased cytokine production shifts the ratio in favor of catabolism—more protein is broken down than is synthesized. The result? Excessive protein losses from the muscle and organ tissues. Many of the people we see remark that it feels like their muscles are melting away. They may in fact be correct. That is why you must eat a high-protein diet and exercise regularly—both will slow muscle wasting.

Fish oil is being studied to see if it can curb the release of cytokines. By reducing the number of cytokines being produced, we think we might ultimately reduce wasting. There is evidence that it works in animals, disease-free volunteers, and people with cancer and other critical illnesses. Our first experiment with people with HIV infection was not successful: cytokines tended to go up. However, we plan to repeat the study using a different fish oil. Other scientists have proposed using pentoxifylline, a drug that blocks the release of one of the cytokines (TNF). These studies have produced mixed results, and work continues. (More on muscle wasting in Chapter 2.)

HYPERMETABOLISM—The HIV infection also causes hypermetabolism. This means that even at rest, you will probably need more calories and burn more calories than someone of comparable height, weight, age, and sex who has no HIV infection. How many extra calories will you need? That depends on the extent of disease. A group of Dutch investigators found that in HIV-infected patients without malnutrition, calorie needs increased by 8 percent. By the way, in this particular study, patients did not lose any weight because they were already eating 500 calories per day beyond their needs. This more than compensated for the 8 percent increase in metabolism.

While the Dutch study looked at HIV infection without malnourishment, a group of French investigators studied the metabolism of people with HIV-infection who were malnourished. And, on average, they found that more calories than normal were needed. However, looking at each patient individually rather than at a group average, the researchers found that 32 percent of the patients either had the same calorie needs as normal or had lower calorie needs. The remaining 68 percent had increased calorie needs in the face of disease. Thus, not everyone needs more calories when they have HIV infection.

Calorie needs also vary greatly with activity level. Many people who in theory are hypermetabolic—but are inactive—do not lose weight. But don't be tempted to sit around doing nothing so that you won't lose weight. On the contrary, if you keep active, your muscles won't further diminish and you'll feel better. (Information on the benefits of exercise, including practical tips and guidelines, starts on page 33.)

Dr. Grunfeld and colleagues did one of the most definitive studies on hypermetabolism causing weight loss in HIV infection. They assessed weight loss due to insufficient calorie intake during a short period and found that malnourished patients with HIV infection had an 11 percent increase in calorie needs. A 154-pound man would need to eat an extra 157 calories daily to avoid weight loss. In people with AIDS, calorie needs increased 25 percent. A person would need to eat an extra 361 calories daily to prevent weight loss. The good news is, both groups of study participants could eat enough extra calories to prevent weight loss during the study.

The third group studied were people living with AIDS who had a secondary infection. Their daily caloric needs increased 29 percent, which meant eating 427 extra calories to avoid weight loss. This demand seemed to be too much, though, and patients lost weight during the study. Ironically, this group ate the fewest calories during the study, although they needed the most. It appears that these patients were anorectic. The anorexia was due to the dual problem of HIV infection and a secondary infection, each of which caused an increase in cytokine release.

This observation emphasizes a unique situation seen in AIDS: frequent secondary infections produce anorexia, which is coupled with increased calorie needs due to hypermetabolism. Together, these conditions lead to weight loss. It is likely that the number of secondary infections in part determines the degree of weight loss, and thus the degree of malnutrition. Unfortunately, this situation may be a vicious cycle, because the more malnourished you are, the more likely a secondary infection will develop. And as the disease progresses, the number of secondary infections increases proportionately with malnutrition. Still, specific steps can and should be taken to delay or minimize any serious complications. And it starts with evaluating your diet and, most likely, changing it to counteract the effects of HIV infection.

Summary

Malnutrition is a common but serious problem for people with HIV infection. It is caused by three factors: loss of appetite, malabsorption, and changes in how the body processes food.

You can become malnourished even if you eat the same foods in the same amounts as before your diagnosis. That means you need to make some changes in your diet to delay or minimize malnutrition. Your first and best strategy is to follow the Principles of Positive Nutrition, which we cover next.

principles of positive nutrition

The most important thing you can do today is change how you think about your diet. So, forget the Basic Four Food Groups and the Food Guide Pyramid you may have seen; you now have different needs.

It's time to learn some new nutrition basics—principles that apply specifically to people with HIV infection. For instance, did you know that very few foods are bad for you? There's even no reason to limit your consumption of foods with high saturated fat and cholesterol. Most people with HIV infection develop low serum cholesterol levels, usually when they are diagnosed with AIDS. We don't know why, but as the disease progresses, cholesterol levels decline. Because of this, high-fat, protein-rich foods can and should be an important part of your diet. In fact, one of the Positive Nutrition goals is to eat twice the normal amount of protein each day.

In this chapter we will fully explain the three Principles of Positive Nutrition. The Positive Nutrition Pyramid will be introduced and compared with the U.S. Department of Agriculture's Food Guide Pyramid. We'll follow that by showing you how to meet your nutrition requirements for calories, protein, fat, carbohydrates, and fluids—even if you are a vegetarian. We'll end with a discussion on how exercise fits into the Positive Nutrition plan.

Your Nutritional Requirements

There are two kinds of nutrients: macronutrients and micronutrients. Macronutrients are calories from proteins, fats, and carbohydrates. (Water is also a macronutrient, but it has no calories.) Macronutrients are not large nutrients as their name implies; rather they are required in larger quantities by the body than micronutrients, which are vitamins and minerals.

Each day, you need to think about how you are going to meet your need for both kinds of nutrients. However, because macronutrients are needed in larger amounts, they require more attention and planning than micronutrients. Many of our patients proudly tell us that every day they take a multivitamin and several single-nutrient pills such as vitamin C and E. While these are important, they contain no calories. Macronutrients contain the calories you need, so a good diet must focus on macronutrients to prevent weight loss.

Scientists know a lot about macronutrients and their role for people with HIV infection. Unfortunately, there's a lot of misinformation out there. Our patients tell us that one of their most frustrating problems is trying to put into practice what they learn from us. Our advice is simple enough, but their friends and caregivers try to impose nutrition rules that apply to themselves but are not appropriate for people with HIV infection. A good example pertains to the fact that all people with HIV infection eventually develop low serum cholesterol levels. Again, we don't know why this happens, but it is probably due to the way the HIV virus affects fats stored in the body. At any rate, people with HIV infection can safely eat the foods with high saturated fat and cholesterol that their uninfected friends should limit in their diet. In fact, as soon after diagnosis as possible, you should make these foods a regular part of your diet because you need them for their high-protein content and for calories to maintain weight. And for your sake, politely disregard the advice of those not knowledgeable about nutrition and HIV infection.

Our Principles of Positive Nutrition are based on published scientific literature and our experience with hundreds of patients. They embody the issues we found ourselves stressing again and again in nutrition counseling sessions. Use these principles to direct your thinking about nutrition, and the thinking of those who care for you.

{principles of positive nutrition}

1. Decide each day how you are going to meet your macronutrient needs (protein, fat, carbohydrates) and spend less time on how you are going to meet your micronutrient needs (vitamins, minerals).
The most severe symptom of malnutrition in people with HIV infection is weight loss, and it is related to macronutrient deficiencies, not micronutrient deficiencies. Macronutrients supply calories; micronutrients do not. This is the most important principle. Give it a high priority, and it won't be hard to achieve.

2. Ignore advertisements, bulletins, and articles aimed at the general public that trumpet information on healthy eating.
General nutrition information may be fine for most but it is not appropriate for people with HIV infection. It may even distract you from achieving your food goals. Very few foods are bad for you. Sugar is all right (and will not encourage the growth of mouth yeast like thrush). Salt is fine, whether it is added at the table or contained in processed foods. Red meat, saturated fats, and dairy products are fine and we encourage their consumption. Avoid foods that present a contamination risk, especially raw fish (including sushi), raw meat, and raw eggs; unprocessed honey and maple sugar; and leftover foods more than 2 days old.

3. Follow a daily meal plan based on the Positive Nutrition Pyramid.
Resolve to make the following your daily food goals—consume:
+ *Twice the normal amount of protein daily (this means 100 to 120 grams for men, 80 to 100 grams for women; 1 pound of meat, poultry, or fish contains about 110 grams of protein)*
+ *At least 2 servings of fruit (1 piece = 1 serving) and 3 servings of vegetables (1/2 cup, cooked or raw = 1 serving)*
+ *At least 2 servings of milk (8 ounces each)*
+ *Enough other calories from carbohydrate and fat to keep your weight stable*

The first Principle of Positive Nutrition emphasizes the need for macronutrients because calories from carbohydrate and fat are vital for maintaining your weight.

{daily macronutrient needs}

CALORIES	15 to 20 per pound of body weight
PROTEIN	Men: 100 to 120 grams of protein
	Women: 80 to 100 grams of protein
FAT	At least 50 grams
CARBOHYDRATES	As much as possible
FLUIDS	The *Positive Nutrition* plan will provide you adequate fluids, with about half coming from beverages, such as milk, juice, and soup, and the other half from solid foods, such as fruits and vegetables. Specifically, you need a 1/2 ounce of fluid per pound of body weight.

Protein and Muscle Wasting

One of the consequences of having HIV infection, or any other infection, is that your body tends to lose muscle. It happens with cancer, also. From the first day you are infected with HIV, this process of muscle wasting occurs. The body actually breaks down its own stores of protein.

Everyone needs a supply of protein each day; the body needs so much that it cannot store enough for the long term. Normally, the body manufactures proteins and breaks down proteins on an equal basis (see page 11). It appears that cytokines released during HIV infection and other infections change this process, causing more protein to be used up than is made. It seems irrational for the body to tear itself apart in the face of disease, but there's a reason: it is something we've inherited from our ancestors.

Let's say that one of our caveman relatives was injured while on a hunt and was not found for days. During that time, he had no food. But to heal, the body needs protein; and our body is designed to be self-healing, with the muscle serving as a source of that protein. At the same time, the body fat is a reservoir of calories that is needed in times of fasting. Thus, the caveman could survive off his own body; using his fat for calories and his muscle for protein. Nowadays, food is plentiful and the supply consistent, so we no longer need to "auto-cannibalize" to survive. But our caveman physiology has not altered over the years; we still use up body protein when an infection or injury is present.

While muscle wasting can be explained, it is still perplexing. A group of German investigators discovered that people in the early stages of HIV infection begin to show signs of muscle wasting even before they lose weight. You would think that if someone lost muscle weight, surely it would

> *To heal, the body needs protein; and our body is designed to be self-healing, with the muscle serving as a source of that protein.*

show up on the bathroom scale—unless, of course, something replaced the muscle. In fact, that's what happens; water replaces muscle.

Using a sophisticated device called bioelectrical impedance, the researchers sent a low voltage current through patients' bodies to measure the amounts of muscle, fat, and water. They found that there was a decrease in muscle weight but a proportionate increase in water weight. The net effect? No change in body weight. Only by use of this device are these subtle differences detected.

We have conducted a similar study at Deaconess Hospital and confirmed these findings. It is only after a person develops AIDS that the body fat weight and body weight will begin to decrease. This loss of body fat occurs usually in response to a poor appetite or anorexia (see Chapter 1).

The best thing you can do to minimize muscle wasting is to eat a diet with twice the usual protein intake and exercise regularly. This won't stop the muscle wasting process completely, but it will slow it down with no added risk to you. On the other hand, if you don't eat enough protein or exercise, the muscles will surely waste faster.

The combination of a high-protein diet and exercise is vital because muscle wasting (and the loss of organ tissue mass), along with general weight loss, are related to the timing of death from HIV infection. Dr. Donald Kotler and colleagues of New York City found that their patients with AIDS died when muscle and organ mass were 54 percent of normal. Weight loss to 66 percent of normal also resulted in death. This is because the body does not have enough strength to carry out necessary functions, such as breathing, making blood cells, and even allowing the brain to work properly and orchestrate all of the body's processes.

As we said, we suspect that cytokines are involved in the body's process of destroying its own muscle stores. Perhaps the body is looking for particular proteins to make new white blood cells to fight off the HIV infection. If so, all the more reason to eat a high-protein diet to give your body more than enough of a variety of proteins to choose from.

{high-protein foods}

FOOD	AMOUNT	APPROX. GRAMS PROTEIN
Meat (beef, poultry, veal, pork, lamb, etc.)	1 ounce	7 g
Milk, soy milk, yogurt (any amount of fat)	1 cup	8 g
Egg	1	6 g
Cottage cheese (any amount of fat)	1/4 cup	7 g
Tofu	1/4 pound	7 g
Legumes (peas, chick peas, lentils, soy beans)	1/2 cup	7 g

Of all of the challenges associated with eating, many people find it hardest to meet their new high-protein goal. Let's face it, 100 grams of protein each day is a lot. And if you don't feel great and are told that you need to eat a big chunk of beef, you're not going to do it with zeal. Fortunately, meeting your new protein goals can be quite easy. The key is to eat protein at every meal and snack so that you portion out your intake throughout the day.

If you are having trouble meeting your protein needs with everyday meals and snacks, you may want to use oral supplements, which we discuss in Chapter 6. Another idea is to combine protein-rich foods with common ingredients (see Chapter 7). Finally, you can try some high-protein recipes in Chapter 8.

Again, because of the virus's effect on the body's muscle, we can't guarantee that a high-protein diet will prevent muscle wasting. But we are absolutely sure that not taking the prescribed protein will exacerbate muscle wasting. And since there is no risk in eating a high-protein diet, and it can slow muscle wasting, we see only benefits in taking it. There are no disadvantages. Remember that your protein needs are twice what is normal; by meeting them, you contribute greatly to your nutritional management.

Fat Facts and Fiction

Your requirements for fat go neither up nor down because you have HIV infection. Still, dietary fat is important for you because it is rich in calories. Even so, you may find that you now poorly tolerate conventional fats. Many people wrongly believe this means that no fat should be eaten because it worsens diarrhea. They avoid fat altogether and lose weight.

The truth of the matter is that there *are* fats that do not cause or worsen diarrhea. As you learned in Chapter 1, medium-chain triglycerides (MCT fats) are absorbed more easily than other fats, making them a sensible alternative for people with HIV infection. HIV infection disrupts normal food absorption, and fats are the hardest foods to digest. The MCT fats contain the about same calories as other fats (9 calories per gram). They are tasteless and odorless and can be used in cooking. MCT fats are not usually available in supermarkets, but are found in most health food stores.

Another myth propagated by some patients is that cholesterol and saturated fats are bad for them. This is categorically false. Much research has been done on the topic, and we and others have found that saturated fats have no influence on immune function. These fats are also rich in cholesterol, which your body needs because HIV infection lowers blood cholesterol. Here, too, resist the conventional wisdom and don't shy away from saturated fats (usually found in high-protein foods), because they are rich in calories.

Unlike saturated fats, vegetable oils that we commonly consume, such as corn, safflower, and soybean oils, do affect immune function.

Research has shown over and over that some vegetable oils suppress the action of the immune system, making it less effective.

So why, then, is our food supply based so much on these oils? Well, one reason is that only vegetable oils contain the two essential fats your body needs every day. Without them, your skin would get very dry, your hair would get brittle, and other subtle changes would occur in your blood cells. We need a little vegetable oil in the diet—about 2 to 3 teaspoonsful each day. Moreover, we need fat to supply extra calories and make foods taste good.

So the question is, how can you get enough essential fats and calories without decreasing immunity? We suggest that you eat oils that are low in immuno-suppressing properties. At home, use butter instead of margarine, and olive and canola oils instead of other vegetable oils. (Olive oil and canola oil are rich in monounsaturated fatty acids, while most other vegetable oils are rich in polyunsaturated fatty acids.) Make this change, and then you can eat the other oils when you go out to eat. This way, you'll get enough essential fats and calories, and support your immune function to the best of our current knowledge.

Fluid Needs

Fluids are especially important to people with HIV infection. A rule of thumb is that you need about 1/2 ounce daily per pound of body weight, if you don't have unusual losses such as with diarrhea. Any fluid counts: coffee, soda, juices, soups, and, of course, water. If you're having trouble keeping up your weight, though, we don't recommend taking non-caloric drinks, including water. Fluids tend to fill you up, so every sip should be useful and contain some calories. Fluid needs during diarrhea will be discussed in Chapter 5. Another area that warrants discussion is alcohol consumption.

Remember, alcohol contains 7 calories per gram (1 gram =1/30 of an ounce; the alcohol content varies widely among different alcoholic beverages). This is more than either carbohydrates or protein. From that point of view, you can have alcohol. But there are two problems with overconsuming alcohol for HIV-infected people. First, alcohol has no other nutritional value. This doesn't matter, though, if you have been following the Principles of Positive

Nutrition, because your body won't need extra nutrients; it will need only calories. Second, alcohol dehydrates you—it removes the water from your blood. If you already have a hard time getting enough fluids, it's best to avoid too much alcohol because it will make the job of staying well hydrated harder.

Pyramid Power

The Positive Nutrition Pyramid should now become your guide to daily eating. It shows six food groups and the minimum servings of each a person with HIV infection should try to eat each day. By following a meal plan based on the Positive Nutrition Pyramid you will meet all of your daily protein requirement and get most of the other nutrients you need. Even so, you'll probably require additional calories, so after consuming the recommended number of servings

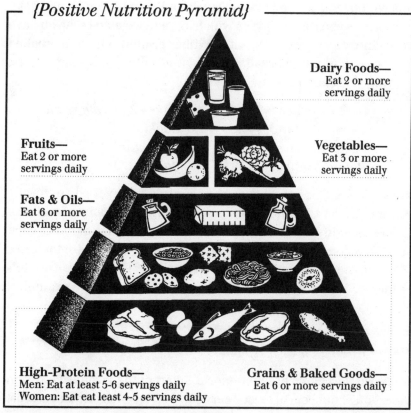

{Positive Nutrition Pyramid}

Dairy Foods—
Eat 2 or more servings daily

Fruits—
Eat 2 or more servings daily

Vegetables—
Eat 3 or more servings daily

Fats & Oils—
Eat 6 or more servings daily

High-Protein Foods—
Men: Eat at least 5-6 servings daily
Women: Eat eat least 4-5 servings daily

Grains & Baked Goods—
Eat 6 or more servings daily

for the six food groups, load up on more foods—from the Pyramid or not—such as cakes, cookies, and ice cream.

The High-Protein Foods group forms the foundation of the Positive Nutrition Pyramid. High-protein foods such as meat, poultry, fish, and eggs are vital for people with HIV infection because they minimize muscle wasting (see also page 18). Men should eat at least 5 to 6, 3-ounce servings each day and women should eat at least 4 to 5 servings. If you are fat intolerant, you should only bake or broil meat, and use no sauces. Serving examples, include:

> *Beef, poultry, lamb,*
> *pork, fish, and*
> *organ meats - 3 ounces*
> *Eggs - 3*

Grains & Baked Goods represent a good source of calories and macronutrients in the Positive Nutrition Pyramid. You should eat 6 or more servings each day. As with fruits and vegetables, if you have gastrointestinal problems, eat low-fiber grain products and baked goods, such as white bread, biscuits, and saltine or soda crackers. Serving size examples, include:

> *Bread - 1 slice*   *Cake - 2-in. square piece*
> *Cereal - 1/4 to 3/4 cup*   *Cookies - 2*
> *Pasta and rice - 1/2 cup*   *Doughnut - 1*
> *Potato - 1/2 medium*   *Bagel - 1/2*

Added Fats & Oils are next on the Pyramid. Many foods naturally contain fats and oils; however, you should make a point of adding 6 or more servings of butter, olive oil, or canola oil to your meals each day. We recommend these specific fats and oils because of their low immuno-suppressing properties (see page 22). If you are fat intolerant, see the section on MCT fats, page 21. Serving size examples:

> *Butter - 1 teaspoon*
> *Olive oil - 1 teaspoon*
> *Canola oil - 1 teaspoon*

Fruits and Vegetables are an important part of the Positive Nutrition plan. You should eat at least 2 servings of fruit each day and at least

3 servings of vegetables. If you have gastrointestinal problems, avoid raw fruit (except bananas) and eat lower-fiber canned fruits, such as peaches and pears. You should also avoid raw vegetables, eating instead lower-fiber canned, frozen, or cooked vegetables, such as winter squash and carrots. Serving size examples, include:

> *Apple, banana, orange, etc. - 1 medium*
> *Raw or canned - 1/2 cup*
> *Juice - 3/4 cup*

> *Cooked vegetables - 1/2 cup*
> *Leafy, raw - 1 cup*
> *Nonleafy, raw - 1/2 cup*

Dairy Foods occupy the top of the Positive Nutrition Pyramid. Your goal should be to eat at least 2 servings of dairy foods each day. If you are lactose intolerant, use lactose-free dairy products and check labels for hidden sources of lactose. Because getting enough calories is so important for people with HIV infection, you should not concern yourself with eating lower-fat products—unless you are fat intolerant, in which case you should use low-fat dairy products. (Read on for more on lactose intolerance; see page 21 for fat intolerance.) Serving size examples, include:

> *Milk - 1 cup*
> *Cheese - 1.5 to 2 ounces*
> *Yogurt - 8 ounces*
> *Cottage cheese - 1/2 cup*

Many people with HIV infection have been told by a doctor or dietitian that they have lactose intolerance. Lactose is a sugar found in all milk and dairy products. Lactose levels vary—there is a lot in milk and somewhat less in fattier dairy products such as ice cream, cheese, and heavy cream (see page 26). People with lactose intolerance lack the protein in the intestine that helps them digest the lactose in milk. The "intolerance" appears as diarrhea, cramping, and bloating several hours after taking such a food; however, the severity of the symptoms varies greatly. (Interestingly, the intolerance to lactose may come and go, so you may want to try a milk product periodically to see whether you are still intolerant.)

{dairy foods' lactose content}

Food	Lactose per 8-ounce serving
whole milk	11 g
skim milk	12 g
regular yogurt*	11 g
low-fat yogurt*	15 g
sour cream	5 tablespoons

Yogurt contains lactase, the protein that breaks up the lactose sugar, so the total lactose content may be less than shown here. Test different yogurts to see whether you tolerate them; individuals respond differently. Frozen yogurt contains no lactase, so it will likely be poorly tolerated. Also test cheeses and creamed soups, which contain varying amounts. Do this on a day you plan to spend at home.

Your doctor can test whether you are lactose intolerant. However, we suggest that if you do have diarrhea, simply avoid lactose-containing foods until it clears up. Then try something like yogurt or aged cheese, which are low in lactose, to see whether the intolerance has passed—remember, it comes and goes. Then graduate to foods that are richer in lactose, such as milk and cottage cheese.

We suggest drinking lactose-free low-fat milk, soy milk, or milk containing acidophilus. These shouldn't cause you any lactose problems and will satisfy your dairy requirements. Or, you can buy a product called Lactaid, which contains the protein needed to digest lactose. Lactaid comes as a liquid or capsule. For more information, call 800-LACTAID. By the way, if you drink Carnation Instant Breakfast, use two doses of Lactaid—one to remove the lactose from the milk and the second to remove the lactose from the powder.

A Pyramid Comparison

The Principles of Positive Nutrition stress that people with HIV infection should ignore nutrition advice aimed at the general public. As a point of reference, we present the USDA's Food Guide Pyramid, which puts much less emphasis on high-protein foods, in particular. This is the appropriate approach for the general public, but it is not right for you. If you compare the two pyramids you'll quickly see how different your priorities must be.

{Positive Nutrition Pyramid}

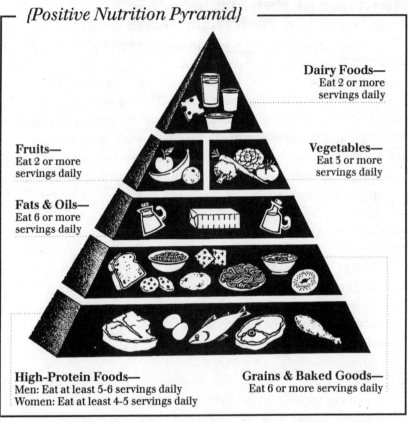

Dairy Foods—
Eat 2 or more servings daily

Fruits—
Eat 2 or more servings daily

Vegetables—
Eat 3 or more servings daily

Fats & Oils—
Eat 6 or more servings daily

High-Protein Foods—
Men: Eat at least 5-6 servings daily
Women: Eat at least 4-5 servings daily

Grains & Baked Goods—
Eat 6 or more servings daily

{USDA Food Guide Pyramid}

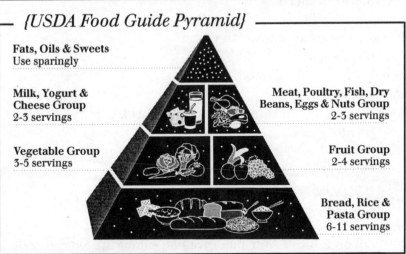

Fats, Oils & Sweets
Use sparingly

Milk, Yogurt & Cheese Group
2-3 servings

Meat, Poultry, Fish, Dry Beans, Eggs & Nuts Group
2-3 servings

Vegetable Group
3-5 servings

Fruit Group
2-4 servings

Bread, Rice & Pasta Group
6-11 servings

How to Meet Your Nutritional Requirements— The Positive Nutrition Meal Plan

If you have been reading this book straight through, you already know the Principles of Positive Nutrition, and you know how many calories and how much protein you need each day. Now it's time to put this knowledge into practice. The following is an overview of a daily meal plan that incorporates all the Principles of Positive Nutrition and the Positive Nutrition Pyramid. The amounts given are the daily minimum; you may certainly have more. You'll also need more calories from other foods, such as snack foods, desserts, and so-called "junk foods."

BREAKFAST
Option 1:

> 1 cup cereal/1 cup milk
> 1 fruit (1 piece, or 1/2 cup)
> 2 toasts or 1 bagel
> butter or cream cheese
> coffee or tea

Option 2:

> 2-3 eggs, not left soft (with cheese, vegetables, optional)
> 3 pieces of bacon
> 2 toasts or 1 bagel
> butter or cream cheese
> coffee or tea

LUNCH

> 6-8 ounces of meat (cold cuts, cooked beef, poultry, pork, veal, lamb, or fish)
> 2 breads, 1 roll, or 1 cup pasta, potato, or rice
> 1 cup vegetables (raw or cooked)
> 2 scoops ice cream*

* Not on Positive Nutrition Pyramid; eat for the extra calories.

DINNER

    6-8 ounces meat (cold cuts, cooked beef, poultry, pork, veal, lamb, or fish)

    2 breads, 1 roll, or 1-2 cups of pasta, potato, or rice

    1 cup vegetables (raw or cooked)

    1 piece lemon meringue pie*

SNACK

    1 cup of milk or yogurt

    2 fruits (2 pieces)

    5 chocolate chip cookies*

* Not on Positive Nutrition Pyramid; eat for the extra calories.

As you can see, the meal plans for lunch and dinner are identical. Needless to say, if the food is prepared the same way as well, you'll get bored pretty quickly. Fortunately, there are countless ways of preparing these meals. In Chapter 7, we describe how to beat the boredom and still get a healthy diet. Enjoy a change of pace by teaming different meats with essential ingredients and optional ingredients. The meats serve as vehicles to carry other tasty components, and by mixing things up, you'll end up with a great variety.

Of course, you can also eat things that don't appear in the meal plan. You may like a stir-fry meat and vegetable medley, spaghetti and meatballs, or tuna noodle casserole. All of these mixtures and many others fit into the plan. Just be sure to start out with about 8 to 10 ounces of raw meat to satisfy the 6- to 8-ounce goal for cooked meat. You may even want to buy a small scale. After a couple of times, you'll get the hang of things—you'll be able to accurately eyeball the correct portion size before you know it.

Even if you eat everything on the meal plan and follow the Positive Nutrition Pyramid, you won't get enough calories to keep your current weight, much less gain weight. Therefore, once you've met your primary nutritional needs for protein and the like, you need to eat other foods. Reward yourself with cookies and milk, chips and dip, pizza, pastries, nuts, or anything you fancy. Most of these foods are the so-called "junk foods," with lots of calories and fat and few other nutrients. If you follow the Positive Nutrition plan, though, you'll meet all your nutritional needs, so you are entitled to reward your self with something frivolous. Foods are "junk" only if they become a substitute for foods on the Pyramid.

Vegetarian Diet

Some people with HIV infection are vegetarians and others want to eat vegetarian meals occasionally, just for variety. Since protein is the vital for your diet, it is important that you still get enough of it without eating its most abundant source, meat. Only meat (beef, poultry, lamb, veal, pork, and fish), milk, and eggs contain all the protein sub-units (amino acids) in the exact amounts humans need.

It is nearly impossible for people with HIV infection who are strict vegetarians to acquire enough high-quality protein in their diet. Very large amounts of dairy products and eggs are necessary. You can, however, get additional protein from legumes, such as black-eyed peas and green peas; peanuts; beans such as soy, kidney, white, black, lima; and lentils. The best protein comes from eating one of these legumes with a grain—such as corn tortilla, rolled oats, rice, bread, or pasta—at the same sitting. The legumes and grains each contain protein; neither has enough amino acids to support the human body, but what is missing from the legume is contained in the grain, and vice versa. But eating legumes for lunch and bread a few hours later does not give the body a high-quality protein; if the two aren't eaten together, the body receives two poor-quality proteins instead of one high-quality one.

The following is a quick reference guide to vegetarian eating. (Remember, women need about 80 to 100 grams of protein every day, men need 100 to 120 grams, and that every ounce of meat contains 7 grams of protein.)

{where to get 7 grams of protein}

FOOD	AMOUNT
beans and peas	1/3 to 1/2 cup
cottage cheese	1/4 cup
cheese, any kind	1 ounce
tofu	1/4 pound
milk or yogurt	1 cup

If you follow a vegetarian diet you need to eat more food to achieve protein goals. For example, 16 ounces of beans supplies only 28 grams of protein, whereas 16 ounces of meat yields 112 grams of protein. Since most people need about 100 grams of protein per day, it will take far more vegetarian food to satisfy the goal. Here is a vegetarian meal plan that meets the Positive Nutrition daily protein goal:

BREAKFAST
>   3 eggs with 1 ounce cheese
>   2 toasts or 1 bagel
>   1 orange
>   coffee or tea
>   1 cup milk

LUNCH
>   1 cup beans
>   1 cup peas
>   1 cup rice
>   1/2 bagel
>   1 apple

SNACK
>   1 cup milk
>   1/3 cup peanuts

DINNER
>   1 pound tofu
>   1 cup salad
>   1/2 cup cooked carrots

As you can see, enormous portions of some of the foods are called for. Eating this much may be difficult, particularly if your appetite is poor. Here's the bottom line: a vegetarian diet is fine in terms of nutrition, but you'll meet your protein needs more easily by eating meat.

Calories: Who's Counting?

We expect that you have some idea what a calorie is. Calories come from only four food sources: fat, which supplies the most calories per gram; carbohydrate and protein, which each provide about half as many; and alcohol, which provides fewer calories than fat but more than carbohydrate and protein. This is shown in the following table:

{food groups providing calories}

FAT	CARBOHYDRATE	PROTEIN	ALCOHOL
9 calories	4	4	7

Everyone—with or without HIV infection—needs 15 to 20 calories per pound of body weight daily. The exact number of calories is mainly determined by how much exercise you do. Go to the gym three or four times a week and you'll need more calories than someone of the same height, weight, and sex who does not exercise regularly. (More on exercise later in this chapter.)

But does the mere presence of HIV infection mean you'll need more calories? In most cases, the answer is no. You do not need more calories simply because you have HIV infection; you're probably already eating enough. However, when you have a secondary infection, such as pneumocystis carinii pneumonia (PCP), you will need a few extra calories—about 400 to 500 more per day. In reality, though, we have seen that on days when our patients have PCP, their activity level drops off. This compensates to some extent for the extra calories required. But if a little weight is lost rapidly, we found that a person's weight can usually be restored quickly after the secondary infection if he or she resumes eating their normal diet.

When it comes down to it, counting calories is probably just an unnecessary worry for you. That's right. The main thing is to eat enough to keep your weight stable, and you'll do that if you concentrate on the Principles of Positive Nutrition and select foods according to the Positive Nutrition Pyramid outlined earlier. Again, the hypothalamus is the section the brain that regulates our caloric consumption; it can work properly even in the presence of HIV infection. If you were at a good weight before the infection, then you should eat enough to remain at that weight.

Many of our patients are slim, and may even be below what is considered normal according to "ideal body weight" tables. But slim people are not malnourished merely because their usual comfortable weight is leaner than most. In fact, we purposely did not include "ideal weight" tables in this book. They only cause undue anxiety.

We have also counseled people with HIV infection who are overweight. For them, we do not recommend active dieting. It is just too difficult to meet the high-protein needs (see Protein and Muscle Wasting, page 18). Plus, active dieting is dangerous because it leads to muscle wasting. Instead, we recommend just eating foods on the Positive Nutrition Pyramid earlier in this chapter.

If you are overweight, resolve to cut back on foods that supply calories but have no nutritive value; that will be enough to induce a slow weight loss without causing any nutrient deficiencies. Most of the overweight people we see opt to eat in this way, skip empty calories, and take part in an exercise program. This is a healthier approach and less risky.

Exercise Your Health

Exercise is as important to you as good eating. Time after time, we see that the active person who exercises maintains muscle and feels the best. It's tougher to manage your exercise than your eating, though. You have to eat, you don't have to exercise.

What can exercise do for you? The benefits of exercise are many, including: increased strength, increased cardiovascular or aerobic fitness, increased flexibility, increased energy, decreased stress, increased lean muscle mass, increased self-esteem, increased confidence, improved sleep, and improved ability to perform everyday activities. With the appropriate guidance and introduction to exercise, you can experience all of these wonderful benefits.

Devise an Exercise Program

To get the most from an exercise program, it is important that you receive proper instruction from a reputable fitness expert, such as an exercise physiologist, physical therapist, exercise specialist, or certified personal trainer. Ask your health care team for recommendations. Clinics and doctor's offices often have a physical therapist or exercise physiologist on staff. (Exercise specialists and personal trainers are more likely to work in health clubs and gyms.) Friends, too, may have suggestions. When it comes to exercise, though, many people think they "know it all," so finding the appropriate professionals to advise you is all the more important.

Once you've identified qualified professionals, meet with them and ask about their background and experience. Make sure you feel comfortable and safe with the individual. The person you choose should assess your exercise needs and devise a personalized program for you. Have your doctor evaluate the program, then find out if he or she wants to continue monitoring it.

+ + + + + + + + + + + + + + + +

Ideally, you should incorporate three components of exercise: cardiovascular fitness, flexibility, and muscular strength.

+ + + + + + + + + + + + + + + +

With HIV infection, you should get regular, moderate exercise. What is moderate? Some people say it is strolling around the neighborhood with the dog. Others consider it nothing less than exhausting themselves at the club. Actually, it is somewhere in between, although the exact level differs from person to person.

Determining an appropriate and safe level of activity starts with knowing your heart rate.

To determine your heart rate, first locate your pulse. To do this, there are two methods: 1) simply place your index and middle finger on the inside part of either wrist; or 2) locate the left or right side of your carotid artery (next to the larynx or voice box) with the same two fingers and apply light pressure to the area. If you feel a rhythmic beating sensation, you have found your pulse. Use a clock with a second hand or have a friend assist you and count the number of beats in 10 seconds. Take that number and multiply it by 6 (or count the beats for 1 minute); this will give you your heart rate.

Calculating your heart rate while at rest provides your resting heart rate (RHR). Once you have done that, you can figure what your heart rate should be while exercising—your "training heart rate." The easiest way to compute this figure is to use the Karvonen

Formula, which uses resting heart rate (RHR) and maximal heart rate (MHR). Normally, this formula is based on a person exercising at 50 to 85 percent of his or her maximal heart rate; however, for people with HIV infection, we recommend using 25 to 50 percent in the formula. Simple calculations to determine your individual "training heart zone" are as follows:

1) Maximal Heart Rate (MHR) = 220 - age
2) Karvonen Formula or Training Heart Rate = (MHR - RHR x .25 to .50) + RHR (beats per minute at 25 to 50% MHR or pulse rate within training zone)

For example:
1) MHR =220-30 (age)=190
2) (190 - 50 x .25 to .50) + 50 = 85 to 120 beats per minute at 25 to 50% MHR

We recommend that you perform aerobic exercise 3 to 5 times per week, with each session lasting 15 minutes to 1 hour. How you feel should determine the amount of exercise you do. Always listen to your body to determine your personal limits of exercise. Some days you may be able to exercise for 45 minutes; other days it may be 15 minutes. The quality of exercise is more important than the quantity!

Ideally, you should combine three components to exercise: cardiovascular fitness, flexibility, and muscular strength. All of these must be part of your fitness program to gain maximal benefit. It's much like the body needing all of the essential nutrients in order to optimize health. Unlike food, we can survive without exercise; however, to optimize fitness health, cardiovascular fitness, flexibility, and muscular strength are essential.

Cardiovascular Fitness

Cardiovascular fitness or aerobic exercise is necessary for a strong heart. Some examples of cardiovascular fitness are walking, running, biking, swimming, and in-line skating. If you find yourself breathing heavy while walking with a friend or climbing stairs, you will benefit from an aerobic training program. If you have other medical issues such as anemia, asthma, or pulmonary disease—for example, a history of pneumocystis carinii pneumonia (PCP)—consult with your doctor before engaging in aerobic activity. The main purpose of beginning a cardiovascular program is to make walking or climbing the stairs less difficult to do. The stronger your heart, the easier these daily tasks will be.

To gain the most from your cardiovascular program, it is important to train within your training zone (25 to 50 percent of your maximal heart rate). After doing aerobic exercise, check your pulse rate periodically over the next 10 to 15 minutes. If your pulse rate is too low (below 25 percent maximal heart rate), you may need to exercise with more intensity. If it is too high (above 50 percent), your body is telling you to slow down. For instance, using the earlier example, the individual should have a pulse rate of 85 beats per minute if working aerobically at 25 percent of maximal heart rate. If the intensity is increased up to 120 beats per minute, then 50% of MHR is achieved.

Flexibility

As important as it is to exercise the heart, it is equally important to improve muscular flexibility. Once you've enjoyed some biking, walking, or jogging, the body must be "stretched out" to prevent muscle soreness and reduce the chances of injury. Neglecting to stretch also means missing out on what is often the most relaxing and enjoyable part of an exercise program.

Stretching techniques, including those for specific muscle groups, are best learned from a fitness expert. In general, though, to maximize flexibility, the stretching should take place after the body has been warmed up with aerobic exercise. In addition, holding each stretch for 15 to 30 seconds rather than bouncing will allow the muscle to easily loosen.

Muscular Strength

The final component of the "total fitness" workout—the development of muscular strength and endurance—is also the most important for the person with HIV infection because of muscle wasting.

There is no evidence that strength training will reverse the effects of wasting; however, a steady strength training program will likely delay its progression.

The development of muscular strength and endurance is based on a theory called the "overload principle." This means that strength, endurance, and size of a muscle will increase only when the muscle is brought to a point of fatigue. In other words, you have to work a muscle before it grows or gets stronger. Because of this, the resistance or amount of weight lifted against the muscle should increase as strength and endurance increases.

Isotonic weight-training is the most common method of strength training. This involves the use of dumbbells, barbells, pulleys, specialized weight equipment such as Nautilus, and also push-up and sit-up like exercises.

Strength training requires gentle progression to prevent soreness and possible injury. Each exercise should include repetitions that are slow and controlled until reaching a point of fatigue. Proper positioning and body mechanics should also be practiced throughout the training program, as well as allowing time for warm-up and cool-down.

You should condition the major muscle groups at least twice a week using a combination of 6 to 10 different exercises with 4 to 8 repetitions each. Results will soon follow with the appropriate regimen designed for you.

Summary

With HIV infection, you have different nutritional needs than the general public. For example, a low-fat, low-cholesterol diet is not suitable for you. Instead, focus on the Principles of Positive Nutrition and develop a daily meal plan based on the Positive Nutrition Pyramid (both shown again on page 38).

The Positive Nutrition approach to eating will help you maintain your weight. And with exercise, it will also minimize muscle wasting and help you stay fit. These two key aspects of your life— appropriate meals and an exercise program—require some effort on your part. But they are areas where you can take matters in hand and make a noticeable contribution to your well-being.

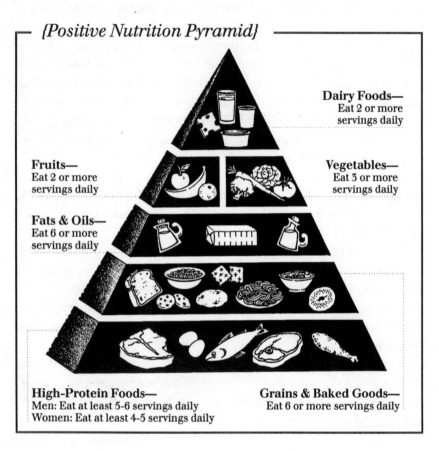

{Positive Nutrition Pyramid}

Dairy Foods—
Eat 2 or more
servings daily

Fruits—
Eat 2 or more
servings daily

Vegetables—
Eat 3 or more
servings daily

Fats & Oils—
Eat 6 or more
servings daily

High-Protein Foods—
Men: Eat at least 5-6 servings daily
Women: Eat at least 4-5 servings daily

Grains & Baked Goods—
Eat 6 or more servings daily

{Principles of Positive Nutrition}

1. Decide each day how you are going to meet your macronutrient needs (protein, fat, carbohydrates) and spend less time on how you are going to meet your micronutrient needs (vitamins, minerals).

2. Ignore advertisements, bulletins, and articles aimed at the general public that trumpet information on healthy eating.

3. Follow a daily meal plan based on the Positive Nutrition Pyramid.

vitamins and other supplements

Doing what's best and avoiding quackery

Many people have unrealistic expectations about vitamin pills and other supplements. Pills cannot and should not replace food. That being said, we do not discount the merits of taking certain vitamin and mineral supplements. In fact, you may need supplements of single nutrients or groups of nutrients to treat deficiencies or to prevent them. The key is first making sure the extra nutrients "do no harm," and secondly, that they may be of some benefit.

Vitamins and minerals are micronutrients. In addition to macronutrients (protein, fat, carbohydrates, and water), micronutrients represent the other source of nourishment everyone needs. In this chapter we will cover which micronutrients are needed in the face of HIV infection. We will teach you how to choose the correct multivitamin and other nutrients that are of potential benefit. And because there has been a lot of misinformation concerning the role of supplements in the treatment of HIV infection, we'll also show you how to spot quacks or quack products.

As always, your focus should be on exercising and getting the proper macronutrients and micronutrients through a Positive Nutrition approach to eating. We have found in our nutrition counseling that while many people worry about getting enough of the necessary vitamins and minerals, few actually accomplish this, even with a multivitamin supplement. A pill will not meet all of your nutritional needs. Nonetheless, supplements are beneficial for many people. Just make sure your information about supplements comes from reputable sources.

RDA's and Positive Nutrition

The Recommended Dietary Allowance (RDA) table on page 42 lists the micronutrients that are required for life and the quantity needed every day. Don't worry, we won't ask you to memorize the table, but you should become familiar with it. The RDAs, set by the National Research Council, are determined by a group of scientists who conduct nutrition research and establish what doses will prevent deficiencies in the general public.

So how do the RDAs apply to you? Many of our patients believe that their nutrient needs are greater because of the infection and because of diarrhea. Our answer is always the same: as far as we know today, the RDA table represents the best and safest guidelines we have for determining micronutrient needs during health and disease. By the same token, depending upon the disease, the RDAs should be modified. And this applies to HIV infection, too.

The Positive Nutrition meal plan presented in Chapter 2 for people with HIV infection provides 100 percent of each of the nutrients in the RDA table. So if you follow our Principles of Positive Nutrition, you'll meet your RDA needs. Nonetheless, we recommend that all patients take a multivitamin supplement, which provides another 100 percent of the RDAs for all vitamins, the mineral iron, and other nutrients such as zinc and iodine.

The vitamin pill you select should also contain a safe and recommended amount of trace elements like manganese, chromium, copper, and molybdenum. A generic multivitamin pill that copies Centrum®, or Centrum itself, is ideal. In essence, if you follow the Positive Nutrition diet plus take a multivitamin pill, you'll get twice the RDA: once from foods and once from the pill. There is no harm in this approach, and it offers more assurance that deficiencies will not arise if there is ever a shortfall in your diet.

You have probably noticed the many so-called "high-potency

multivitamin/multimineral pills" that are available. Surprisingly, some contain 1,000 percent of the RDA of some vitamins but lack other essential nutrients found in the RDA table. Usually, these pills are rich in B-complex vitamins, because they are inexpensive. Excess B-vitamins are excreted in the urine and cannot harm you. However, more costly trace elements, such as selenium, are often omitted. Thus, not only are the supplies of some nutrients inadequate, but megadoses of others are provided, which , depending on formulation, may disrupt the required balance of micronutrients in the diet. We therefore suggest that you choose multivitamin pills that contain 100 percent of each nutrient on the RDA table, which follows.

> *Surprisingly, some high-potency multivitamin/multimineral pillscontain 1,000 percent of the RDA of some vitamins but lack other essential nutrients.*

For some essential nutrients, no RDA has been established; instead, a range is given called the Estimated Safe and Adequate Daily Dietary Intake of Additional Selected Nutrients. If you are now taking vitamin and mineral supplements, we suggest that you use this table to compare with the supplement label. Remember, 100 percent of most of these nutrients is all you need. Are you taking more than that?

Vitamin Supplements: What's Safe, What's Not

Vitamins are one of two types: water soluble and fat soluble. Water-soluble vitamins (the B vitamins and vitamin C) are constantly being used up or excreted in urine, so they need to be replaced each day. On the other hand, fat-soluble vitamins such as vitamin A, D, and E are absorbed in fat and stored in the fat tissue. Because of this, they can build up to toxic levels if too much is consumed.

Vitamin E is needed to protect the fat housed around your blood cells by not allowing the fat to become rancid. It also works as an antioxidant. Antioxidants are helpful because they can neutralize harmful oxygen or oxygen-containing components that circulate in

{recommended dietary allowances}
(ages 23 to 50)

NUTRIENT	MEN	WOMEN
Vitamins:		
A	1,000 mcg RE*	800 mcg RE*
Thiamin (mg)	1.4 mg	1.1 mg
Riboflavin (mg)	1.7 mg	1.3 mg
Niacin	19 mg equiv.[†]	15 mg equiv.[†]
C (mg)	60 mg	60 mg
D (micrograms)[‡]	5 mcg	5 mcg
E (mg; 1 mg = 1 I.U.)	10 mg	8 mg
K	80 mcg	65 mcg
Folic acid (micrograms)	200 mcg	180 mcg
B6 (mg)	2.0 mg	1.6 mg
B12 (micrograms)	2.0 mcg	2.0 mcg
Minerals:		
Iron (mg)	10 mg	15 mg
Calcium (mg)	800 mg	800 mg
Magnesium (mg)	350 mg	280 mg
Phosphorus (mg)	800 mg	800 mg
Trace Elements:		
Zinc (mg)	15 mg	12 mg
Iodine (micrograms)	150 mcg	150 mcg
Selenium (micrograms)	70 mcg	55 mcg

No RDA has been established for the following essential nutrients—
Estimated safe and adequate daily dietary intake:

Chromium (mcg)	50-200 mcg	50-200 mcg
Copper (mg)	1.5-3.0 mg	1.5-3.0 mg
Manganese (mg)	2.0-5.0 mg	2.0-5.0 mg
Molybdenum (mcg)	75-250 mcg	75-250 mcg
Fluoride (mg)	1.5-4.0 mg	1.5-4.0 mg
Vitamin K (micrograms)	70-140 mcg	17-140 mcg
Biotin (micrograms)	30-100 mcg	30-100 mcg
Pantothenic Acid (mg)	4-7 mg	4-7 mg

*retinol equivalents: 1 R.E. = 5 international units (I.U.)
[†]mg equivalents: 60 mg of tryptophan = 1 equivalent
[‡]mcg: 100 I.U. = 2.5 micrograms

the blood in response to cell damage. The toxicity dose of vitamin E has not yet been determined but intakes of 10 times the RDA appear safe.

In contrast, vitamin A and D approach a toxic level at doses above twice the RDA. In fact, the law requires that all vitamin pills contain no more than 100 percent of vitamin D per daily dose. Vitamin D, which promotes calcium absorption for healthy bones and teeth, is found in milk and milk products such as cheese. It also comes from exposure to sunlight.

Vitamin A promotes good vision and maintains healthy skin, teeth, and skeletal tissue; it is highly toxic, though. Many centuries ago, Eskimos ate polar bear liver as a delicacy. The story goes that death occurred almost instantly after eating the liver. It didn't take long to see that this was a bad idea. Later, scientists found that polar bear liver contains the highest concentration of vitamin A of all mammalian tissues. Most vitamin pills today contain modest amounts of vitamin A, but taking too many multivitamin pills will provide too much of it. Instead, choose a safe, nontoxic alternative to vitamin A: beta carotene, which the body converts to vitamin A in a controlled fashion and only when needed.

Two reputable investigations have been published concerning the use of multivitamin supplements by people with HIV infection. One was conducted with 296 HIV-infected patients in San Francisco (Abrams, AIDS, 6:949-958, 1993); the other was done in Baltimore and included 281 patients (Tang, *American Journal of Epidemiology*, 138:937-951, 1993). Both studies determined that in people with HIV infection who took multivitamin supplements, the progression to AIDS was slower than in those who didn't take the supplements. This makes sense on the surface because generally most people who take better care of themselves by eating health-fully, taking prescribed medications, and visiting their physician also regularly take multivitamins.

What isn't clear from either report is why some vitamins and minerals seemed to slow the progression to AIDS and others sped it up. For example, in the California study, iron, vitamin E, and riboflavin appeared to retard the progression. But in the Baltimore study, the highest intakes of vitamin C and thiamin appeared to slow it. Also, it appeared that those who took the most vitamin A, niacin, and zinc had an increased rate of progression to AIDS. We still don't fully understand these results; however, as more studies are done it is conceivable that a special vitamin for people with HIV infection will need to be made. Meanwhile, you'll do best if you take a multivitamin that meets 100 percent of all the nutrients on the RDA table and eat a healthy diet.

Megadoses of single nutrients should be taken with caution, but there are a few that hold promise. If you decide to take some extra vitamins, we recommend three antioxidants that have been studied extensively: vitamins C and E and beta carotene. To review, antioxidants can curb the damaging effects of harmful oxygen or oxygen-containing components in the blood. Extensive research has been done at Tufts University in Boston on these nutrients and their effect on immune function in the elderly, chosen because immune function declines with age. Since HIV infection can cause cell damage, we think that vitamins C and E and beta carotene supplements may be appropriate for you. The initial results are promising, and taking them won't hurt you.

In addition to a healthy diet and a multivitamin, we recommend that you take the following amounts of these selected antioxidants. This applies whether you have HIV infection or have been diagnosed with AIDS.

{recommended dietary supplements}
(for males and females)

vitamin C	500 to 1,000 mg
vitamin E	10 to 40 International units (I.U.)
beta carotene	6 mg (10,000 I.U. of vitamin A)

Our reading also suggests that the above nutrients not only may boost your immune system but also may have an additional benefit. First, several studies show that beta carotene levels in the blood decline during AIDS. Beta carotene is absorbed only with fat, and if fat is poorly absorbed, beta carotene may be also poorly absorbed. Thus, supplemental beta carotene may allow blood levels to remain normal. Second, vitamin E levels are usually normal in people living with AIDS or HIV infection, although it too needs to be absorbed with fat. As mentioned earlier, vitamin E protects the fat around your blood cells. Basically, this fat becomes rancid if too little vitamin E is around, and preliminary evidence shows this is true in people with HIV infection. So, although vitamin E intake may seem to be normal, the additional amount from a supplement may be beneficial.

There is not much published directly about the benefits of vitamin C for people with HIV infection. However, as an antioxidant, vitamin C may protect blood cell membranes. Therefore, we think you should take it in addition to vitamin E and beta carotene.

Higher doses of vitamin E and beta carotene have been shown to enhance immune function without producing side effects; however, at present we suggest these modest doses. Note that selenium is also an antioxidant, but you'll get all you need from a multivitamin tablet. Never take it as a single nutrient; it is extremely toxic.

Mineral Supplements: What's Safe, What's Not

Like vitamins, certain minerals are essential for life, including calcium, phosphorus, magnesium and iron. (All are listed on the RDA table.) You won't benefit from taking excesses of any of these unless you have a deficiency.

Extraordinary amounts of calcium, magnesium, and phosphorus may be lost when diarrhea exceeds one quart a day for more than seven days. However, the biggest problem is not with overdosing but with taking in insufficient amounts of these essential nutrients. For example, we found that about half of our patients drink no milk. It is nearly impossible to get enough calcium, magnesium, and phosphorus without consuming two cups of milk or yogurt each day. As we will discuss in Chapter 5, if milk is poorly tolerated, lactose-free, low-fat milk can be substituted; it contains the same amount of calcium, magnesium, and phosphorus as regular milk.

If you absolutely can't or won't take milk or yogurt, we suggest eating cheese, cottage cheese, soy milk, or even sardines every day. In addition, you would be wise to take four regular or three extra-strength TUMS, or the same dose in a generic equivalent. Phosphorus is abundant in all processed foods and sodas, so don't worry about getting enough of it. Magnesium is found in cereal grains, green vegetables, seafood, and nuts—so eat more of these foods. Don't take magnesium supplements unless your doctor finds that your blood magnesium is low, because these irritate the gastrointestinal tract and can cause diarrhea.

Iron is needed daily and comes primarily from meats, fish, and poultry. Foods such as dried raisins and beans contain some iron, but it is in a form that the body does not absorb well. Iron is needed by the red blood cells to help carry oxygen, which gives you energy. Iron deficiency anemia is common during HIV infection, and your doctor may order iron supplements if the iron level in your blood is low. Don't take iron on its own without a physician's order except in a multivitamin; it irritates the intestine and may cause constipation.

While mineral deficiencies are less well-documented than vitamins, current knowledge suggests that a healthy diet is sufficient to avoid mineral deficiencies.

While mineral deficiencies are less well-documented than vitamin deficiencies, current knowledge again suggests that a healthy diet is sufficient to avoid mineral deficiencies. Thus, your multivitamin pill need not contain calcium, magnesium, or phosphorus.

Trace Element Supplementation: What's Safe, What's Not

Look again at the RDA table (page 42) and you'll notice that among the trace elements, only selenium, zinc, and iodine have RDA values; the remaining trace elements should be supplemented according to the estimated safe range.

In general, trace elements should not be taken individually for two reasons. First, many are toxic in surprisingly small doses. Second, they are required in precise balances that occur naturally in foods, and supplementation of one may create an artificial deficiency of the other. For example, excessive zinc supplementation can lead to copper deficiencies. Thus, we suggest you take a multivitamin that contains the trace elements listed in the amounts shown in the RDA table.

Much attention has focused on the role of selenium in HIV infection. This is because selenium is an antioxidant and appears to slow the rate at which the HIV infection spreads in a group of cells in a test tube. However, we don't know what dose a person needs to get this beneficial effect. We do know that more than double the RDA of selenium can be extremely toxic, so despite the promising results in cell culture, humans are limited to this dose. It is likely that you are best off with the safe dose of selenium found in many multivitamin and mineral pills plus the other antioxidants listed earlier.

Herbs, Glutamine, and Other Supplements: What's Safe, What's Not

The least studied but perhaps most promising supplements are herbal preparations and other nutrients often found outside the mainstream of conventional medicine. Since there is little scientific support for using most of these nontraditional preparations during HIV infection, we cannot advocate many at this time. At present, studies are under way in our laboratory on the use of ginseng to boost immune function.

Two nutritive agents that do not appear on the RDA, yet hold some promise in the near future for people living with AIDS, are glutamine and N-acylcysteine (NAC).

Glutamine is an amino acid (used to make protein) made by your body. If you are not in perfect health, the body cannot make enough of it; there is also evidence that the body needs more glutamine during illness. Dr. Douglas Wilmore, a physician at Harvard Medical School, and colleagues, reported that cancer patients who had bone marrow transplants and received glutamine had fewer infections than a group who didn't take glutamine. Recently, the same investigators found that other patients with chronic diarrhea who needed total parenteral nutrition (TPN) because they couldn't absorb conventional foods also benefitted from glutamine. These patients had fewer bowel movements and could eat a regular diet again. Many didn't need TPN anymore. In addition to supplemental glutamine, the patients received fiber and growth hormone.

Dr. Wilmore's group also found that people with AIDS have abnormally low levels of glutamine in the blood. Supplementation with 20 grams of glutamine each day failed to return the blood level to normal. Studies are under way to determine whether 40-gram doses are adequate.

To learn more about glutamine, we suggest you read *The Ultimate Nutrient: Glutamine* by Judy Shabert, MD (Avery Publishing Group, Garden City Park, NY, 1994). The author has studied glutamine with her husband, Dr. Wilmore. She delves into such topics as the role of glutamine in improving immune function, improving muscle mass, and healing the digestive tract. In addition, we have referred several patients to a clinic near Boston that uses this approach. For more information, call the Nutritional Restart Center at (800) 867-6761.

There are also some promising studies on NAC (N-acylcysteine), but most have been done in the laboratory, not the body. L-NAC (not the D-form) could be used to correct a deficiency of glutathione, which inhibits HIV infection replication. Interestingly, glutathione is made up of glutamate, which comes from glutamine. There may be a relationship between glutamine and NAC; however, clinical studies are inconclusive and no dose has been established, so speak to your doctor before taking L-NAC or glutamine.

> *Growth hormone and anabolic drugs promote muscle development and may prevent wasting. However, the action of both growth hormone and anabolic drugs is short term—once you stop using them, the benefits disappear.*

The only other related treatments that are actively being studied and have shown some promise are growth hormone and other anabolic drugs. In fact, at Deaconess Hospital we are currently studying their potential benefits for people with AIDS. Growth hormone and anabolic drugs promote muscle development and may prevent wasting. Unfortunately, growth hormone is expensive and may have side effects. The anabolic agent oxandrolone, which we are studying, is relatively inexpensive. However, the action times of both growth hormone and anabolic drugs may be short term—once you stop using them, the benefits may disappear.

We again suggest you take the Positive Nutrition approach of eating a healthy diet and exercising regularly. There is some evidence to suggest that testosterone or oxandrolone would be a suitable substitute for growth hormone. Testosterone is a male hormone responsible, in part, for muscle development and is often depleted in people with AIDS. However, it has side effects, specifically mood changes. Preliminary evidence suggests that oxandrolone causes fewer side effects. Most prescription anabolic drugs, coupled with a good diet and exercise, may be safer and less costly than growth hormone, and may be equally effective in maintaining muscle mass.

Although glutamine, NAC, and anabolic agents appear promising, more work is needed before any will be routinely recommended by physicians working with people with HIV infection. We discussed the therapies because they represent three examples of high-quality research work being done in the area of HIV infection and AIDS. Again, before you take supplements not prescribed by your doctor, consider what the product does, its side effects, and its proper dose.

How to Spot Quacks or Quack Products

Anyone with a serious disease can be an easy target for hucksters selling just about anything claiming to eradicate disease and make users feel better. People with cancer and AIDS are most often approached by these unscrupulous vendors. We know, because we hear it from our patients. It's also evident when we speak to large groups about the merits of Positive Nutrition. More often than not we are assaulted by people who want us to use their products or allow our names to be used in their promotions.

The problem with quacks or quack products is that very likely none of them work. Let's face it, if something were that good, your doctor would know about it and prescribe it. Some quack therapies may even do you harm. The Food and Drug Administration (FDA) is thinking of requiring warning labels on some foods such as herbal teas and aloe, which contain stimulant laxatives which pose health risks to many individuals. Some teas containing senna have led to adverse reactions, including diarrhea and cramps.

Use following guidelines when considering these therapies—or anything not recommended by your doctor, nurse, dietitian, or other conventional health care professional.

Evaluating Alternative Therapies and Products

1. Is there a sound scientific basis for seeking nonconventional care and products? To make sure a treatment is effective, it must undergo rigorous scientific testing. Of course, this frustrates many people because it takes a long time to conduct studies properly. The FDA has attempted to speed up this process for AIDS-related drugs and therapies. Nonetheless, you would never take a drug from your doctor without knowing that it works. The same standards should apply to nonconventional therapies.

2. Is the product safe? Are there recommended doses on the package? Do you know anyone else that has taken the product? Most of the dietary supplements sold in the United States are safe. All are regulated by the FDA. Unfortunately, the regulation is limited to safety, not how it works. Thus, no one at the FDA will claim that a dietary supplement is effective, but they will state that the product is safe. In reality, the only time these products come to the FDA's attention is when someone gets sick or dies after use. You may remember the incident involving L-tryptophan, an amino acid that was alleged to alleviate depression and help people sleep better. It wasn't the L-tryptophan that caused people to become sick; rather, it was caused by unsafe production methods by a single manufacturer.

If you are using a dietary supplement, at the first sign of any adverse side effect, stop taking it immediately. If you are taking multiple supplements, you should stop them all and re-introduce them one at a time. This is the procedure your doctor would follow if there were adverse side effects from a conventional drug.

3. Did a knowledgeable person advise you about the therapy? The best recommendations come from physicians and other health care professionals. And use your common sense. If it's too good to be true, it probably is.

4. Are the supposed results so dramatic that you are instantly hooked into taking the product? Be wary of supplements that claim to eradicate HIV infection, cure wasting, or get rid of all secondary infections. These are complicated problems, and the best treatments are those prescribed by your doctor. If you wish to try such alternative products, do so, but always in conjunction with drugs prescribed by your doctor. Be sure to tell your doctor about all the supplements you are taking because there may be undesirable interactions between the prescribed drugs and non-prescribed supplements.

Tell your doctor about all the supplements you are taking because there may be undesirable interactions between the prescribed drugs and non-prescribed supplements.

5. Is the manufacturer of the therapy reputable? Always determine who the manufacturer is. You may want to call the company about a product you are considering and ask about their manufacturing practices. Ask if the FDA has recently inspected their manufacturing facilities and request a copy of a written report of the visit.

In one single copy of a newsletter written for people with HIV infection, we noted that 8 of the 23 pages were devoted to the merits of castor oil. No results of this treatment appeared in reputable journals. However, one study claimed that topical application of castor oil packs increased T-pan lymphocyte counts (T-11), but there was no evidence that patients experienced fewer secondary infections or lived longer. There were also several anecdotal remarks by patients and a statement that more information is available from the company selling the treatment. These data do not appear compelling enough to warrant widespread use of this therapy. Other examples of alternative therapies should be viewed in the same way.

Summary

By following the Principles of Positive Nutrition, you'll receive the Recommended Dietary Allowances for vitamins and minerals. Nonetheless, we recommend that you take a multivitamin supplement, which provides another 100 percent of the RDAS for all vitamins, the mineral iron, and other nutrients such as zinc and iodine. It should also contain a safe and recommended amount of trace elements like manganese, chromium, copper, and selenium. By taking a multivitamin each day, you'll get twice the RDA: once from foods and once from the pill.

In addition, we recommend that you take these additional supplements: vitamin C (500 to 1,000 mg), vitamin E (10 to 40 I.U.), and beta carotene (6 mg). Overdosing of other single nutrients is not necessary and may be harmful.

As for herbs and other nontraditional supplements, we cannot advocate many at this time. More research must be done before any nontraditional therapy will be routinely recommended by physicians working with people with HIV infection. Many of our patients are eager to explore alternative therapies. This is fine, but you must take steps to ensure that the alternatives don't interfere with conventional treatments or have undesirable side effects.

tests and measurements— working with your doctor

No one knows your health and how you feel better than you. You know if you haven't been very hungry lately. You know if you've had problems with diarrhea. Or you know if you're feeling better than ever. The key is using that insight as a starting point to improved care. In this chapter, you'll get the necessary tools to do so. You'll learn the specific health indicators you should track. Then, we'll show how to use this information to work effectively with your doctor and get the tests and support you deserve.

Where Do You Stand Nutritionally?

Changes in your health can occur so gradually that they're hard to recognize from day to day or even month to month. For instance, it may be months before you realize you have been slowly losing weight. However, by recording specific aspects of your health (your weight, in this case), you can detect changes early and always keep ahead of the game.

Certain medical tests and measurements are key indicators of your health and nutritional status. In the sample chart on page 56, we provide the framework for assessing your nutritional health and keeping ongoing records. (Copy it as needed for additional assessment charts.) The goal is to detect changes early, so it's important to obtain and record specific information at least every 6 months. Then, with your doctor or dietitian, you can head off or minimize any problems.

All of our proactive patients keep records of their medical information. Whether you are an avid record keeper or not, this is an important tool in taking control of your health and in tracking your nutritional information. If you can't stand recordkeeping, "appoint" a friend to the job. It's that important.

Your nutritional assessment starts with measurements of your weight, preferably using the same scale each time, and your waist size. Don't worry if your weight falls out of the "normal" range according to an ideal body weight table; your nutritional status can be judged only in relation to your starting weight. Keep in mind, though, if a 5-pound weight loss does occurred, go to your physician; if you wait until you've lost 20 pounds, it may be difficult or impossible to do anything about it.

Besides body weight and waist size, certain blood tests may show improvement in response to proper eating plans, or at least no deterioration. Set up a schedule with your doctor for measuring the serum albumin, triglycerides, and cholesterol every 6 months when your routine blood samples are taken. These blood tests are good indicators of nutritional status: as the status worsens, triglycerides rise and the other values decline. Your goal should be the following values:

Blood Test Goals

+ *Albumin—above 3.2 g/dL*
+ *Cholesterol—above 100 mg%*
+ *Triglycerides—below 1,000 mg%*

Don't worry if your albumin level suddenly falls; it will do that if you have a secondary infection when the blood is taken, no matter what your nutritional status is. If your albumin is measured again 3 weeks after the infection goes away, it should be where it was before the previous reading.

Body measurements and blood tests don't tell the whole story, though. You'll also need to record your appetite, aspects of your bowel habits, any secondary infections and cancers, and hospitalizations during that 6-month period.

For the appetite section, be sure to assign a general level to your appetite and whether you used appetite stimulants during the past 6-month period. Record the product name and dose for future reference. Of course, appetite habits may change briefly, but try to capture the best description of your appetite during the past 6 months.

There are two sections to complete for bowel habits. In the first and second of these, record the number and consistency of stools that you usually have each day. Next, assign a letter to rate your perception of abdominal pain and bloating. Of course, these will vary, but again try to capture a realistic picture of the past 6 months.

Body measurements and blood tests don't tell the whole story. You'll also need to record your appetite, aspects of your bowel habits, any secondary infections and cancers, and hospitalizations.

Finally, in the last sections, record the presence of any new secondary infections or cancers. Also, record there whether you were hospitalized during the last 6 months, and if so, why and for how long.

{6-month nutritional record}

DATE:

weight

waist

CD4 count
(cells/mm3)

viral load
(HIV RNA copies/ml)

albumin
(g/dl)

cholesterol
(mg%)

triglycerides
(mg%)

general appetite: A=yes, good;
B=moderately good;
C=poor (if C, name drug
and dose if you are taking
an appetite stimulant)

diarrhea (usual number
of movements per day)

consistency of stool:
A=formed to hard; B
=soft; C=watery

abdominal pain and
bloating: A=none; B=mild;
C=moderate; D=severe

secondary infections or cancers
(yes, no; if yes, describe nature,
treatment, and duration)

hospitalizations (yes/no;
if yes, nature and duration)

Discussing Weight Loss

It's clear that your weight is a key measurement and therefore an important discussion topic for you and your doctor.

Weight loss may occur for several reasons, as outlined in Chapter 1. The two main treatable reasons are (1) you are eating less, and (2) the loss of nutrients through malabsorption or diarrhea. Treatment is more effective in the early stages, which makes it all the more important that you tell your doctor when you have lost weight, either suddenly or slowly over time. He or she may have noticed the weight loss, but will not necessarily bring it up. It is quite appropriate for you to voice concern about your weight.

As mentioned earlier, weight loss of more than 5 pounds needs to be brought to your doctor's attention. If you don't have a scale but your pants seem baggy or you've moved your belt a notch tighter, that may also be an indication that you should talk to your doctor about your weight. It reflects either a significant change in your appetite or diarrheal losses, or both. It is practically impossible to lose this much weight otherwise; just ask anyone who is trying to diet how difficult it is to lose 5 pounds. It is just as hard for an obese person to lose weight as a person of normal weight.

Your conversation with your doctor about weight loss or any other concern should focus on the problem, so a sensible treatment plan can be devised. In nutritional issues, your main role is to identify problems. The doctor may do so too, but must also assess, diagnose, and treat the problems as early as possible.

Besides raising your nutritional concerns with your physician, you may wish to speak with a registered dietitian. These health care professionals are registered by a national association and trained both in the medical aspects of diseases and in counseling to improve nutritional status. Your doctor or hospital may be able to recommend a dietitian to you. Otherwise,The American Dietetic Association (ADA) at 800-366-1655 can put you in touch with one in your area. The ADA also has a listing of dietitians who specialize in HIV infection, so be sure to ask for this reference specifically.

You might want to visit a dietitian every six months to determine your actual calorie intake and weight. You may also want to review that you are taking appropriate foods for your medical condition. If needed, discuss the use of oral supplements. Dietitians can assess your nutritional status and may relay this information to your doctor. A dietitian can help you with meal planning, and help determine whether or not you are a candidate for a tube feeding diet or total parenteral nutrition (TPN).

The following describes how you might take steps to tackle the two treatable factors that produce weight loss—decreased appetite and increased diarrhea—by raising them with doctors.

Decreased Appetite

When you lose weight because of decreased appetite alone, you'll have to verify that your food intake has changed. You may want to determine with a dietitian what your normal intake used to be, say a year ago, and what your intake is now, and compare the intake to the goals discussed in Chapter 2. The dietitian can calculate the calories and protein consumed then and now. Or you can simply write down the foods that you used to eat during a typical day and those that you eat now; this should enable you and your doctor to determine whether a decreased appetite is causing your weight loss. Anorexia can be treated with appetite stimulants, but your doctor should check whether you have any other problems like diarrhea, which needs to be treated first.

Diarrhea

Many people with HIV infection lose their appetite because of diarrhea—every time they eat they get diarrhea, so they simply eat less. Whether you have diarrhea or just loose bowel movements is a tough call. There are many definitions of diarrhea. Usually, diarrhea involves increases in the number of bowel movements you have a day and in the consistency, where it becomes more liquid-like.

We have found that one of the toughest topics for people to speak to their doctor about is their bowel habits—including the associated pain and changes in stool formation that have occurred. Of course, diarrhea *is* unpleasant and inconvenient, and it may be uncomfortable for you to discuss these issues with anyone, including your doctor. Also, you may wrongly feel that these things are unimportant or of no interest to your doctor. Nonetheless, we strongly urge you to describe in detail all changes that have occurred along your intestinal tract, including changes in your throat, stomach, lower abdomen, and stool. Many of your symptoms are treatable if they are correctly diagnosed. And many times the key to finding the best treatment is figuring out which area of the intestinal tract is affected.

— *{intestinal tract problems}* —————————

AREA OF INTESTINAL TRACT	POSSIBLE SYMPTOMS TO TELL YOUR DOCTOR ABOUT
THROAT/ESOPHAGUS	difficulty swallowing pain/soreness reflux of foods and liquids from stomach
STOMACH	fullness/bloating/gas ...all the time ...during or immediately after meals pain vomiting nausea reflux/burping
INTESTINE	bloating/gas ...all of the time ...during or immediately after meals pain
STOOL/BOWEL MOVEMENTS	diarrhea ...frequency ...consistency ...time of day/pattern constipation/straining

There are numerous tests your doctor can use to find the cause of your complaints. Some tests are simple to perform, non-invasive, inexpensive, and can be done regularly. Others are invasive and costly, and are reserved for severe problems. Usually, though, there is a fine line between complaints your doctor perceives as mild and those he or she perceives as severe. Partly, your doctor bases the decision to use certain tests on the level of concern you express.

You may say, "I have a little diarrhea, but it doesn't bother me because I can still go to the gym and visit my friends without fear of not making it to a bathroom on time." In this case your doctor may prescribe a stool examination for ovum and parasites, and take some blood samples. These could provide a fairly accurate diagnosis of the problem. But don't hold back; if your problems are more severe, say so.

On the other hand, you may come to the doctor and say: "I am very unhappy with the amount of diarrhea that I am having. I don't even want to leave the house. I always get diarrhea after a meal, so I've begun to eat less. I feel weak and can't keep even water inside me sometimes."

You will remember from our discussion of diarrhea in Chapter 2 that either the small intestine or colon (or both) may be impaired, producing severe symptoms. In this case, the doctor will likely take a more aggressive approach, and even perhaps order an endoscopy that could lead to a more precise diagnosis. This involves inserting a long tube into your throat and down into your intestine. The tube has a light at the end so the doctor can look inside to see whether there is any irritation. A small section of your intestine can be taken and sent to a laboratory for analysis of the pathogen. Your intestine can't feel anything, so the biopsy is painless. The worst part of the procedure is when the tube goes down your throat. However, you are given a mild anesthetic, which alleviates the discomfort and makes you forget the unpleasant experience.

Sometimes, depending upon the severity of diarrhea, your doctor may wish to explore whether you are absorbing the foods you eat. Most of these tests involve measurements of your blood and stool. For example, individuals with severe diarrhea may lose fat in their stool. The doctor can order a test called a fecal fat test. If the doctor orders a 72-hour test, the patient collects all of his/her stool over 3 days into a container the size of a paint can. Or the doctor can measure fat from a single stool sample. Patients need to eat a high fat diet during the 3 days and the day that the single stool sample is taken, or the test doesn't work. This is because if just a little fat is eaten, there is less chance that the body will lose any of it in the stool; and the test will show that there is no problem when in fact there may be one. Only by eating a regular diet, rich in fat (as outlined in Chapter 2) to meet your needs, will the test report true fat losses.

Typically, the body will absorb most of the fat in the diet. If more than 5 grams (1/6 of an ounce) appears in the stool, this usually indicates that fat absorption is incomplete. It may be necessary for you to eat a low-fat diet in conjunction with formulas containing MCT fats (see Chapter 6).

People who absorb fat poorly often have trouble absorbing other things, such as vitamins (e.g., beta-carotene, folic acid, and B12), which are measured in the blood. Some people with seriously impaired intestines are unable to absorb complex sugars found in starchy foods. The d-xylose test should show whether this is also a problem.

Therapy for gastrointestinal problems varies but usually includes treatment of (1) the agent causing the problem, which is likely a parasite, bacterium, fungus, virus, or tumor; and (2) the symptoms, such as nausea or diarrhea. Once the agent causing the problem has been identified and the symptoms have been successfully treated, an appetite stimulant can be prescribed.

Tests Your Doctor Can Order

Presented on the next page is a reference table that you can use when you speak with your doctor. It includes some of the tests that can be ordered if you or your doctor suspect that there is a problem with the absorption of nutrients that is causing or could cause malnutrition. Don't hesitate to discuss these tests with your doctor as soon as symptoms appear.

─ *{tests your doctor can order}* ──────────

TEST	WHAT IT MEASURES	REASONS IT IS ORDERED
MACRONUTRIENTS		
FECAL FAT a) 72 hours b) spot test from a single bowel movement	• whether all the fat in the diet is absorbed, • measures fat in the stool	• chronic diarrhea, particularly as a result of a large meal • weight loss
D-XYLOSE	• to check whether all of the complex carbohydrate eaten is absorbed • measures d-xylose in urine and blood	• diarrhea • weight loss
MICRONUTRIENTS		
BETA-CAROTENE	• whether levels in the blood are normal (beta-carotene can be absorbed only when fat is absorbed properly)	• diarrhea • fat malabsorption • weight loss • poor appetite
B12 (SHILLINGS TEST)	• whether levels in the blood are normal (B12 comes mainly from animal products like milk and meats; many vegetarians require regular B12 injections)	• diarrhea • weight loss • poor appetite • vegetarian diets
FOLIC ACID (FOLATE)	• whether levels in the blood are normal	• diarrhea • weight loss • poor appetite

The micronutrient tests shown above are a bellweather in terms of absorption of other fat-soluble vitamins (beta carotene) and of other water-soluble ones (B12 and folate).

If there are problems with the absorption of fat and carbohydrate, the diet may have to be modified to enhance absorption of these nutrients. Special oral supplements may be required. However, if the micronutrient tests are abnormal, no dietary modifications are available. In some cases your doctor may determine that you may need TPN , or prescribe supplements of single nutrients (see Chapter 6).

Summary

Taking charge of your health starts with learning how to judge your nutritional status, so when there's a change you can act quickly to correct it. By using the chart provided in this chapter to track your nutritional health, you'll have the vital records in one place.

Armed with this information, you can speak to your doctor about nutrition-related issues and take proactive measures—measures based on fact not memories that may be less than perfect. Once the appropriate diagnostic tests are ordered and interpreted, both the symptoms and the causes of the problems can be treated. Remember, speak up as soon as symptoms appear—don't wait.

Ask to be referred to a dietitian if you are having trouble sticking to your meal plan, or if you are not tolerating certain foods. Dietitians are trained to give you the help you need and to adapt the Positive Nutrition guidelines to your particular situation.

when you don't feel well

Although most days you will feel well and have a good appetite, there will be days when you feel crummy. Perhaps it's caused by fever, mouth sores, or an irritated throat. Or, you may have stomach or intestinal problems.

When you feel lousy, you probably won't feel like eating. However, your body still needs adequate nutrition on those days.

This chapter begins with some general guidelines for eating when you don't feel so well. Then we move into specifics and offer suggestions about what you should eat when you're facing a particular problem: fever and night sweats, diarrhea, constipation, abdominal bloating and pain, mouth sores and throat pain, or nausea and vomiting. We also will give you some rules of thumb regarding when you should call your doctor.

Guidelines

You should always do your best to follow the Principles of Positive Nutrition (see page 17). However, on days when you don't feel well, treating a specific condition or symptom takes precedence.

We have devised some general "Eating When You Feel Lousy"

tips, which were gathered mainly from our patients and from material written by other health care professionals. We know it's difficult for even the most motivated people to take charge of their nutritional care when they don't feel well. Nonetheless, we hope these tips will help.

When You Feel Lousy

1. Avoid getting dehydrated at all costs. Even when you are well, you need 1/2 ounce of fluid per pound of body weight every day. And if you have a fever or diarrhea or are vomiting, you'll need more fluid still. On average, you'll need two extra cups of fluid a day with a fever or vomiting. If you have diarrhea, you should try to take three or four extra cups.

2. Maintain the minerals in your body. Nutrients such as sodium and potassium are abundant in foods but get depleted quickly during vomiting and diarrhea. If you feel fatigued at these times, it is mainly because of the loss of these minerals. To replace sodium, eat canned soup and bouillon. Potassium can be obtained from fruit juices and nectars.

3. Don't eat or drink too quickly. When you feel crummy—particularly when your stomach and intestine are upset—it's best not to blast your system with foods. Even water, if it is drunk fast, will irritate an already sensitive body. We suggest diluting every calorie-containing beverage such as juice, soda, or nectar with an equal amount of water. Soup, coffee, and tea don't have to be diluted. Chew solid foods thoroughly (it may help to put your fork or spoon down between bites).

4. Avoid the "forbidden" foods. When you feel lousy, certain foods are practically guaranteed to set your stomach or intestine off. Don't worry if you avoid a specific type of food for a few days or even weeks; there are nutritious alternatives, as the following shows.

Forbidden Foods	Substitute Foods
Milk and milk products such as cheese, cottage cheese, and sometimes yogurt; ice cream; frozen yogurt	Lactose-free, low-fat milk and cheese; plain or vanilla yogurt may be OK—try it once to see what happens
Raw fruits and vegetables; any type of gas-producing vegetable (broccoli, cauliflower, Brussels sprouts, cabbage)	Canned fruits without skins or fibrous parts (peaches, pears, melon, bananas); vegetables without skin or seeds (potatoes, winter squash, carrots)
Fried and greasy foods; sauces because they may contain milk	Baked or broiled meats; lean cold cuts (no visible fat); eggs, boiled for at least 10 minutes
Spicy foods (this usually depends on the individual, but be careful of hot curries)	Bland foods
Rich desserts, doughnuts, pastries, beverages	Stewed or canned fruit without skin or seeds, gelatin, sherbet, ice pops; carbonated beverages with sugar, fruit juices or nectars (always dilute with 1/2 water), sports drinks; remember not to drink too quickly
Very hot or very cold foods	Foods cooled or warmed to room temperature (except for frozen desserts)
High-fiber foods such as raw vegetables and fruits, especially those with skins (peas, corn, grapes) or seeds (cucumber, zucchini); whole grain breads	Stewed or canned fruits without skin or seeds; cooked vegetables such as winter squash or carrots; white bread, low-fiber cereals, white pasta, low-fiber crackers, plain bagels, English muffins, white rice; breads and crackers made with white (non-whole grain) flour are the easiest to digest and cause the least intestinal disturbance

5. Call your doctor if severe symptoms persist longer than 3 days. You need the immediate attention of a physician if you have extremely high fever (over 100° F); profuse diarrhea or a major change in the number of bowel movements; or you are vomiting more than two or three times in an hour. Don't wait it out or try to play doctor. Stomach problems, a sore mouth, and other symptoms described in this chapter may indicate that something is wrong, and it is likely to be treatable. By taking some initiative, you can get problems corrected early, which usually results in minimal side effects.

Managing Specific Symptoms

The following pages describe common symptoms people with HIV infection face, as well as the foods that should be eaten—or avoided—for that particular problem. No matter the problem, though, do what you can to keep hydrated and try to eat nutritious foods. Above all, err on the side of contacting your doctor too early rather than too late.

Fever and Night Sweats

Persistent fevers and night sweats are common for many people with HIV infection. Sometimes fever and night sweats are a sign of something serious about to happen, for instance, a bout of PCP (pneumocysistis carinii pneumonia). Many other times, though, nothing happens, or a minor annoyance like the flu or a cold strikes.

Sometimes, the fevers occur at night. You know the feeling: you wake up in the middle of the night covered with sweat. This could occur for weeks and then simply disappear, or it might yield to treatment with something no stronger than aspirin, ibuprofen, or acetaminophen. Call your physician if you have regular fevers so that a decision can be made about testing for the origin of the fever.

No matter what the cause, two things always happen when you have a fever: First, you lose your appetite; and second, your fluid requirements increase.

With a fever, you'll need about 2 extra cups of fluid daily over your normal needs (1/2 ounce per pound of body weight). For instance:

┌─ *{fluid needs}* ─────────────────────────────────────┐

Weight	Normal fluid needs	Extra fluid needs with fever	Total fluid needs
150 pounds	75 ounces (about 9 cups)	16 ounces (2 cups)	91 ounces (about 11 cups)

└──┘

Eleven cups of fluid may seem like a lot, even on a day when you feel well. However, you normally get about half of your fluid in solid foods, where the fluid content is disguised.

On days with fever, we know that you will have less appetite, so you'll likely be taking most of your fluid as beverages rather than iin solid foods. Because of this, we suggest that when you have high fevers (over 100° F), drink a couple of ounces of a caloric beverage, such as a non-diet cola, every 15 minutes. This mimics an intravenous infusion of fluids—but without the needles. Drinking fluids every 15 minutes helps you avoid dehydration, which is the number one rule of the "When You Feel Lousy" guidelines (page 66).

Now let's consider the example of the 150 pound person with fever who isn't eating solid foods. This person needs about 91 ounces of fluid. If 8 hours are set aside for sleeping, 16 hours are left for drinking. To figure this person's fluid intake:

┌─ *{calculating fluid intake}* ─────────────────────────┐

16 hours (awake) x 60 minutes/hour
= 960 minutes during which to drink.

In 960 minutes there are 64 segments
of 15 minutes (960÷15 = 64);

thus, 91 ounces÷64 segments
= 1 1/2 ounces every 15 minutes.

└──┘

It is probably not necessary to be this precise; we merely want to offer you a way to cope with increased fluid needs when you've lost your appetite. This way you'll avoid both dehydration and swamping your intestine with too much fluid too quickly. Of course, if you can eat, you won't need to take this much fluid.

Foods with lots of fluids include fruits, vegetables, soups, Jello, ice cream, and pudding. There is little fluid in meat, bread, and pasta.

Diarrhea

Diarrhea tops the list of most common complaints we hear from our patients. The problem is not continuous diarrhea; rather it's the diarrhea that comes and goes often.

As we discussed in chapter one, malnutrition is caused by the symptoms accompanying diarrhea, not usually by diarrhea itself. For example, one of the first things a person usually does to "treat" diarrhea is to stop eating. This decreases the amount and frequency of diarrhea, but contributes to malnutrition, particularly if the diarrhea persists for a long time.

It's best to aggressively manage diarrhea. Once it is under control, then the diet needs to be modified in various ways. Steps of managing diarrhea are listed below in order of preference. Of course, there are exceptions, but these serve as general guidelines. Most causes of diarrhea can be identified and, even better, treated. Reporting the symptoms to your doctor when you first get diarrhea will permit early treatment, causing you less discomfort and

{anti-diarrheal products}

NAME	OVER-THE-COUNTER (OTC) OR PRESCRIPTION	WHAT IT DOES
Metamucil	OTC, a powder consisting of soluble and insoluble fibers from the husk of psyllium seeds	binds the intestinal fluid so that stool becomes formed
Pepto-Bismol	OTC, liquid or tablets	controls diarrhea, lessens abdominal cramps, and relieves nausea
Imodium	OTC, capsules	slows flow of food in intestine and diminishes fluid loss in the stool
Lomotil	prescription, pill or liquid; may be habit forming, so take only prescribed dose	slows flow of food in intestine and diminishes fluid loss in the stool
DTO (deodorized tincture of opium)	prescription, drops; use only after intestine is clear of pathogen; may be habit-forming and make you groggy	same as Imodium, but stronger
Sandostatin	prescription, injected	reduces the amount of digestive juices formed so diarrhea is less

reducing the chances of malnutrition. The treatments of diarrhea are numerous, so if the first line of attack doesn't work there are many alternatives.

Sometimes, even after undergoing a number of tests, your doctor will not be able to tell you what is causing the diarrhea. This is called "path-negative" (pathogen negative) diarrhea, and we believe that it is really being caused by the HIV infection or by a hidden pathogen. In these cases, it is best to continue taking the antiretroviral medication that treats the HIV infection; this may also treat the "path-negative" diarrhea as well. If a pathogen is identified, you'll need to continue taking your antiretrovirals for HIV infection plus a medicine to treat the "pathogen" or bug that is causing the diarrhea.

Medical Steps to Control Diarrhea

1. Don't wait more than 3 days before calling your doctor. And do not accept the answer, "Well, diarrhea is just part of the disease of HIV infection." As we have described, there may be treatments.

2. Discuss with your doctor how to discover the cause of the diarrhea. Tests may include blood tests, stool tests, and endoscopy, where the gastroenterologist takes samples of the inside of your intestine. Usually, if blood tests identify the problem, no other tests will be needed, and you will be given one or more antibiotics to take for several weeks. Sometimes after finishing the prescribed dose the diarrhea will reappear. Call you doctor immediately. The most likely cause of the diarrhea is the same pathogen as before, and the antibiotic treatment will be extended.

3. Always check with your doctor before using anti-diarrheals, even though some are sold over the counter. These drugs slow the flow of foods and intestinal juices through the intestine. Some anti-diarrheals may be used before a pathogen is identified, some after.

Dietary Steps to Control Diarrhea

1. Keep yourself hydrated. You'll need your maintenance fluids (1/2 oz per pound of body weight) plus another 3 or 4 cups daily, depending upon the number of bowel movements.

2. Keep your blood minerals normal. Due to the large losses of sodium and potassium, you need to replace them aggressively. This is easy. Sodium is obtained from table salt; foods with visible salt on them, such as chips, nuts, and crackers; pickled foods, cold cuts, and canned foods; soups and canned solid meals such as spaghetti. Potassium is obtained from fruits, fruit juices, vegetables, and meats.

3. Select foods that do not exacerbate diarrhea. As we discussed earlier, there are a number of forbidden foods. (For their nutritious substitutes, see page 67.)

{forbidden foods}

Milk and milk products	Rich desserts
Raw fruits and vegetables	Very hot or very cold foods
Fried and greasy foods	High fiber foods
Spicy foods	

Constipation

Constipation does occur during HIV infection, but usually only intermittently after bouts of diarrhea. It may also result from a medication that you are taking. After prolonged periods of severe diarrhea, you can become constipated simply because "there is nothing left to come out." It may also occur because the anti-diarrheal medication has kicked in and slowed your intestinal flow too much. For people with hemorrhoids, the tendency to strain when constipation occurs exacerbates that condition.

One way to avoid constipation is to eat a high fiber diet or a fiber supplement such as Metamucil. This tends to prevent or to treat constipation as well as treat diarrhea. Dehydration also induces constipation, so again, keep well-hydrated.

Usually, though, constipation isn't a chronic condition and treatments should be examined carefully; the last thing you want is to create a diarrhea-like state. Waiting 48 hours for a bowel movement is all right. Beyond that, call your physician and seek out the best treatment.

Abdominal Bloating and Pain

The second most common complaint (after diarrhea) is that of bloating, pain, gas, rumbling—you name it. There is something not right between the stomach and the end of the large intestine. Most of the time it feels as if an army is marching down your entire gastrointestinal tract, pounding as it goes along, and every once in a while punching the sides, causing intermittent discomfort. When the pains aren't severe, some people say it feels as if someone is continually inflating and deflating a balloon in their intestines. There is a constant feeling of fullness and discomfort.

Abdominal bloating and pain nearly always indicate that foreign bacteria have moved into the intestine and ousted the normal bacterial residents. In the large intestine, bacteria live symbiotically next to the cells lining the intestine. Both foreign bacteria and bacteria that normally reside in the large intestine can digest foods that manage to escape your small intestine. Some even produce vitamin K, an essential nutrient that helps blood to clot.

When your immune system is compromised, and especially when you are taking antibiotics, the normal bacteria counts diminish, allowing foreign bacteria to move in and take their place. These invaders and normal bacteria produce a lot of hydrogen gas, which can be measured on your breath. A more bothersome side effect is that the hydrogen gases build up within your intestine and cause a bloated feeling. It is extremely important that you see your doctor within a week of the first symptoms. You will usually need a full blood and stool work-up to identify which bacteria are causing the problem. Most of the bacteria found in the intestines of people infected with HIV can be treated. Thus, there is no reason to delay seeking treatment.

Because of the bloating and feeling of fullness, it is best to eat small, frequent meals. You can eat all kinds of foods, but it is likely that the bacteria will become more active when you eat fruits and vegetables, fried foods, and sometimes milk and milk products—ice cream, cheese, yogurt, and creamed soups and sauces. Fiber-rich foods should be avoided because they cannot be fully digested; they simply migrate into the colon and feed the foreign bacteria. This leads to more bloating and pain. Never take liquids with solid foods because they will fill you up too quickly. It's best to wait half an hour before or after a meal to drink something.

Mouth Sores and Throat Pain

Mouth sores, such as canker sores, and throat pain are also common problems associated with HIV infection and AIDS, as well as the medications related to the disease. Many people also report having "dry mouth." Not only are these conditions a real annoyance when trying to eat, but they may also contribute to dehydration.

The key is to eat or drink nothing that further irritates your mouth and throat. It's important to drink plenty of fluids to avoid dehydration. Many people find that beverages are soothing, especially cold ones such as the Positive Nutrition Shake shown below. Adding gravies and sauces to meats and vegetables may make them easier to eat. Generally, though, avoid tough foods (inexpensive cuts of meat) that may be too chewy. You'll find that softer, moister foods, such as fish, are best. Sticky foods, such as peanut butter, may pose problems and make you feel that you are going to gag.

Canned supplements or making your own high-calorie milk shake can replace a meal and will not irritate your mouth or throat as much as solid food. When you have pain or dryness in your

---

{positive nutrition shake}

Add to a blender and blend well:

1 cup of whole milk or yogurt
1/2 to 1 cup ice cream, sherbet, fruit, or fruit juice.
Any other flavorings or ingredients to taste, such as vanilla, honey, sugar, pasteurized liquid egg, chocolate syrup, and instant pudding mix.

---

mouth or throat, we suggest that you consume at least two canned supplements or shakes each day. The best supplements are reviewed in Chapter 6.

Mouth sores can be readily treated with prescription drugs. Don't wait until you are in extreme pain; contact your doctor within 3 days when you feel there is a problem. You may want to keep the medication on hand to use as needed. Similarly, with throat irritation, contact your doctor early. It is usually easily treated.

Dry mouth, on the other hand, is more difficult to treat, although it is less serious medically. There are several artificial saliva preparations that may offer some relief. The standard advice, though, is to suck on ice chips or candy sour balls. It's best to be taking calories and fluids constantly, so keep a Thermos filled with a milk shake or chilled canned supplement handy to sip on. You should be able to get at least 500 calories from these foods and beverages and make your mouth and throat feel better at the same time.

Nausea and Vomiting

It is nearly impossible to eat when you are nauseated or vomiting. Fortunately, these symptoms pass quickly so there is no need to force yourself to eat.

As always when you aren't feeling well, be sure to keep yourself hydrated, even if it is with a little ginger ale or other carbonated beverage. (Let the carbonation disappear, though, before drinking these sodas.) With a queasy stomach, taking small, frequent sips helps. Keep a glass by your side at all times and sip at least every 10 to 15 minutes. You may also feel like drinking broth, bouillon, or juices. Ideally, if you can tolerate them, drink canned supplements or milk shakes; these provide protein and calories. Remember, you'll need about 2 extra cups of fluid over and above your regular daily fluid needs of 1/2 ounce per pound of body weight.

You can skip solid foods for 24 to 48 hours, but beyond that, you should contact your physician. Some solid foods that go down fairly easily are salted crackers, puddings and yogurt, and warm and cold cereals. Similar to liquids, small, frequent meals of solid foods are best. (Never eat lying flat on your back; always have at least your head and shoulders elevated.)

Just the smell of food may make you feel worse, so stay away from the kitchen. Ask a friend or someone else to prepare food and beverages for you. We also recommend that everyone keep a supply of frozen dinners on hand. They are a great help in avoiding the preparation and lengthy cooking associated with most meals. It is best to buy only entrees that contain at least 20 grams of protein per serving; be sure to read the label on the box. If you are feeling really queasy, you may be better off eating one of the "diet" meals, which are low in fat and calories but high in protein.

Both nausea and vomiting are treatable and should be dealt with by your physician if they are prolonged—more than 2 or 3 days. Sometimes these symptoms are related to a flu that is going around, sometimes to the HIV infection, but most likely to some medication that you are taking. Talk about the symptoms with your physician. There are anti-nausea drugs to prevent vomiting. Or your doctor may change your medication.

Summary

There will be times when you won't feel well. You may not want to eat because of diarrhea, fever, or some other reason. Despite this, you can and should take specific steps to eat and drink what you can and manage the cause of your condition. This may mean putting the Principles of Positive Nutrition on hold temporarily, but you and your doctor should aggressively deal with your symptoms.

In general, when do not feel well:

+ *Consume enough fluids to avoid getting dehydrated.*
+ *Maintain or replace lost nutrients, such as sodium and potassium.*
+ *Don't eat or drink too quickly.*
+ *Avoid "forbidden" foods (see page 67).*
+ *Call your doctor if your symptoms persist more than 3 days*

While the problems described in this chapter can lead to malnutrition, they need not do so. Careful dietary management and working with your doctor can eliminate symptoms early and lower the chances that you will become malnourished.

beyond the Positive Nutrition Pyramid

You may reach a point when it is not possible to keep up with your nutritional needs by eating conventional foods and following the Positive Nutrition Pyramid. For instance, try as you might, you may not want to eat because you just aren't hungry. Or, if your small intestine is badly damaged, foods may be too complex to be absorbed. Whatever the reason, you need to prevent malnutrition, which means you may have to replace or augment everyday foods to obtain optimal nutrition.

You've got several options to maintain or improve your weight: oral supplements that come prepared in cans or "juice box" packages, or those that need mixing; tube feeding diets; and intravenous diets, typically referred to as TPN (total parenteral nutrition). All of these nutrition alternatives are nonexperimental and have been used for over 20 years for a variety of diseases.

Oral supplements are just what their name implies—supplements to the regular diet. If you're not eating anything else, many supplements alone will not provide complete nutrition. However, they can be effective in overcoming diet shortfalls or gastrointestinal problems.

Tube feeding formulas, on the other hand, are complete diets that can nourish a person for years. A feeding tube is either inserted through the nose into the stomach, or directly through the abdominal wall and into the stomach or intestine. Tube feeding is often referred to as enteral nutrition; the word "enteral" means "through the intestine." Some oral supplements are also tube feeding diets.

Intravenous nutrition, called total parenteral nutrition or TPN, is also not experimental. Nutrient-rich solution is administered through a catheter that is placed in a large vein ("parenteral" means "by vein") that flows directly into the heart.

Do You Need an Alternative Diet?

Like other parts of your medical care, you can and should have a big role in selecting the best methods of nourishing yourself. Alternative diets need to be discussed first with your doctor, but you can certainly take the initiative and suggest their use rather than waiting for your doctor to do so.

Choosing the best alternative diet is a two-step process. First, you and your doctor need to establish whether you really need some other form of food. Second, if the answer is yes, it must be determined which is the best alternative diet for you, given your medical condition.

If you have any of the following symptoms, you are likely a good candidate to receive one or more of the alternative diets:

+ *Lack of appetite*
+ *Weight loss of over 5 pounds*
+ *Diarrhea (more than 3 movements per day)*
+ *Altered taste sensations*
+ *Abdominal bloating or cramping*
+ *Depression*
+ *Being treated for an opportunistic infection or tumor*
+ *Generalized fatigue; not feeling well*

The three alternatives to conventional diets are usually tried in order, with oral supplements coming first, tube feeding diets next, and intravenous feeding last. (In fact, insurance companies often will not reimburse the cost of TPN therapy if oral supplements were not tried first.) You may have to skip part of the progression if you obviously need the next level of nutrition. The following table shows when each of the alternative diets should be used. You do not need to have all of the symptoms to be a candidate for a particular diet; rather these items reflect the most prominent reasons for receiving each diet.

These alternatives diets are effective only if you are actively being treated for HIV infection. If at any time you refuse all options of care offered by your doctor, these forms of nutritional support should be discontinued. They simply don't work unless the whole body is receiving therapies.

{alternative diets}

TYPE OF ALTERNATIVE DIET	IF YOU HAVE:
Oral supplements	loss of appetite weight loss (less than 10 pounds) diarrhea (less than 5 movements per day) fatigue lack of interest in food and cooking abdominal bloating/pain
Tube feeding diet	loss of appetite weight loss (more than 10 pounds) diarrhea (5 to 10 movements per day) fatigue lack of interest in food and cooking mouth sores throat pain or soreness
Total parenteral nutrition (TPN)	weight loss (more than 10 pounds) diarrhea (more than 7 to 8 movements per day) confirmation by test that there is malabsorption of fat, fat soluble vitamins, vitamin B12, d-xylose, or protein inability to hydrate self unable to keep up with mineral losses loss of appetite fatigue lack of interest in food and cooking

Oral Liquid Supplements

It is likely that every person with HIV infection will at some point require oral liquid supplements. As mentioned before, these products merely supplement the standard diet; many do not offer complete nutrition.

Oral supplements are a good option at various times because they add a high-quality blend of nutrients to your diet. First, if you have gastrointestinal disturbances such as nausea, bloating, a feeling of fullness, or diarrhea, specific types of supplements will provide extra calories and protein without making your condition worse. Second, supplements are also helpful when you are too busy or tired to eat a proper diet. It is not that you can't eat or won't eat; you just don't have the time or energy to prepare wholesome foods. Last, supplements are often used if you have a poor appetite—you simply don't feel like eating enough to meet the guidelines in the Positive Nutrition Pyramid (page 23).

Over 100 oral supplements are available for people with HIV infection, so it is pointless to attempt to list them all here. Instead, we have grouped them into three categories and provided a few examples of each. The products within each category have a similar composition and, more important, the same use.

STANDARD SUPPLEMENTS

Composition—resembles blenderized foods; contains carbohydrate, protein, fat, vitamins, and minerals

When Used—requires a fully functioning gastrointestinal tract; should be used when lack of appetite is the main problem

MODIFIED FAT SUPPLEMENTS

Composition—usually contains less than 10% fat, if more fat, it is mostly in the form of medium-chain triglycerides (MCTs); protein is either in a form requiring full digestion or broken down into smaller pieces for easier digestion; also contains carbohydrate, vitamins, and minerals

When Used—for people who have diarrhea or other stomach and intestine problems that prevent intake of enough calories and protein

SPECIAL FORMULA SUPPLEMENTS (containing fish oil and a blend of proteins)

Composition—also available in bar form; contains sardine oil and, in liquid form only, a protein broken down into smaller pieces to facilitate absorption, which may help immune function

When Used—for people with general digestion problems and wasting; not use to be used to counteract fat malabsorption (the sardine oil will not be absorbed adequately)

Standard Supplements

Standard supplements—the most common type—contain carbohydrate, protein, and fat in the same form as it appears in conventional foods. This means that you'll need a normally functioning gastrointestinal tract. If you have diarrhea and are sensitive to fat, you shouldn't drink these supplements. But if you lack appetite and have no abdominal pain or diarrhea, these products are perfect for you.

You probably know some of the products in this category. Ensure, Resource, and other standard supplements are sold in cans over the counter in local drugstores and large chain stores such as Walgreens, Kmart, and Wal-Mart. Even Carnation Instant Breakfast qualifies as a standard supplement. For more information about these products, including the possibility of home delivery, contact the manufacturer.

ENSURE (the powder is less expensive than the ready-to-use version), ENSURE PLUS, ENSURE HIGH PROTEIN

Manufacturer—Ross Laboratory, Columbus, OH; 800-227-5767 (nutrition information) or 800-544-7495 (order only)

BOOST, SUSTACAL

Manufacturer—Mead Johnson Nutritionals, Evansville, IN; 800-247-7893 (nutrition and ordering information)

RESOURCE, RESOURCE PLUS

Manufacturer—Sandoz Nutrition, Minneapolis, MN 800-999-9978

CARNATION INSTANT BREAKFAST
Manufacturer—Clintec/Nutrition, Deerfield, IL
800-422-2752 (nutrition information)

MEGAMASS 2000 (a Joe Weider product)
Manufacturer—General Nutrition Center, Pittsburgh, PA
800-274-8558
We tell many patients to try MegaMass 2000 because it contains one of the best protein sources for people with HIV infection. Be wary of any powder or drink that contains a "hydrolyzed" form of casein, whey, or lactalbumin, or that says, "free amino acids added." You'll pay a premium for these items that aren't needed. Again, all the products in this group are appropriate only if you have no problems with digestion.

Modified Fat Supplements
This group of products contains fats that are easier to absorb and less likely to cause or exacerbate diarrhea. Unlike standard supplements, these supplements are complete diets that can replace food on a short-term basis. People with diarrhea, especially those with fat malabsorption, are ideal candidates for these products. Some of our patients with severe diarrhea will take only such modified fat diets for 7 to 10 days to allow the intestine to "cool down." Again, these supplements are for the short term; once the diarrhea clears up, resume a standard supplement.

The products in this category either contain very little fat—just enough to prevent deficiencies—or contain the normal amount but mostly in the form of medium chain triglycerides. MCT fats are extremely easy to digest and absorb. Research has shown that people with AIDS that have severe fat losses lose much less fat when they switch to MCT-rich liquid diets. Some of these products also contain high-quality hydrolyzed proteins, which are digested more easily than proteins left in their natural state. Thus, for people with severe diarrhea, we recommend diets rich in MCT fats and hydrolyzed proteins.

LIPISORB

Manufacturer—Mead Johnson Nutritionals, Evansville, IN
800-247-7893 (nutrition and ordering information)

PEPTAMEN*

Manufacturer—Clintec Nutrition, Deerfield, IL
800-422-2752 (nutrition information)

VIVONEX PLUS[†]

Manufacturer—Sandoz Nutrition, Minneapolis, MN
800-999-9978

VITAL HN*

Manufacturer—Ross Laboratory, Columbus, OH
800-227-5767 (nutrition information) or 800-544-7495 (order only)

*Contains hydrolyzed proteins in addition to modified fat.

[†]Contains amino acids (protein in its purest form) and very little fat.

You or your insurance company will pay a premium for modified fat supplements. But when your gastrointestinal tract isn't functioning, and if you don't tolerate standard supplements, then these are worth the price, especially because their use is short term. Unfortunately, they also taste bad. However, most come with flavor packets and recipe booklets. Be creative, for instance, some people have found that adding Crystal Light or Kool Aid to Vivonex Plus improves it. Nutrition Medical, Inc., (800-569-7828) offers less costly generic versions of Peptamen and Vivonex.

Remember, these modified fat products are useful only when you have a hard time tolerating regular foods and standard supplements. If these don't work, it may be that your intestine is so damaged that intravenous feeding is needed.

Special Formula Supplements

Advera, a liquid supplement from Ross Laboratory, is patented for people with AIDS to combat general digestion problems and wasting. The supplement contains fish oil, one of the most difficult substances to absorb, and hydrolyzed protein. A clinical study conducted in California has shown that two cans of Advera taken daily for 6 months will help decrease the number of hospitalizations and maintain weight better than taking the same amount of one of the standard formulas (Ensure). However, before sanctioning widespread use of a food product or drug, we would generally like to see at least two studies. More work is currently under way.

A mixture almost identical to Advera was made into a bar by NCI Medical Foods. If you are tired of liquid supplements, try the bar. The cost of the liquid and the bars is comparable. A second study is currently underway.

ADVERA
   Manufacturer—Ross Laboratory, Columbus, OH
800 227-5767 (nutrition information) or 800 544-7495 (order only)

NUBAR HIGH CAL
   Manufacturer—NCI Medical Foods, Irwindale, CA
800 869-1515

Tube Feeding Diets

Tube feeding diets are used when the intestine works well enough to absorb what the body needs, but the person cannot or will not take food by mouth. Many cancer patients, for instance, rely on tube feeding diets because food cannot travel in the usual fashion, from mouth to stomach, if a portion of their esophagus has been removed. Tube feeding diets can also be used by people with poor appetites or those who are too tired or sick to eat.

Only a handful of our patients with HIV infection have been good candidates for tube feeding. The reason? If their only problem is a poor appetite, appetite stimulants usually work and they can drink enough of the oral liquid supplements to complement their meals; tube feeding isn't necessary. And those with poorly functioning intestines require a modified-fat supplement described earlier. Beyond that, if the intestine becomes really dysfunctional, intravenous TPN is needed. Still, we encourage their use when appetite is poor and doesn't respond to stimulants, especially since the risks associated with tube feeding diets are very few.

Types of Feeding Tubes

If your doctor has found that you can absorb all the nutrients you need but just can't eat, there are several ways to receive the tube feeding diet. Some of them are invasive; that is, the tube has to be inserted through your skin. Others are not; the tube simply slips through your nose.

Many people learn to insert the tube through their nose every night, receive the formula while they sleep, and remove the tube in the morning. Others leave the tube in place for a couple of months and stay home until they gain a little weight. However, if the tube is left in the nose for too long—about 2 months—the sides of the nose begin to erode. So if you need a long-term feeding tube, it is best to select an invasive one.

There are four major categories or types of feeding tubes:

✦ *A naso-gastric feeding tube is intended for short-term use by a person with no evidence of nausea and vomiting. After the nose is sprayed with a mild numbing agent, a small tube is inserted through the nose into the stomach by a doctor, a nurse, or the patient.*

✦ *A PEG (percutaneous endoscopic gastrostomy) feeding tube is intended for long-term use, also by someone with no evidence of nausea and vomiting. It is inserted by a gastroenterologist, who uses an endoscope to aid the passage of the tube through the abdominal wall. Local anesthesia is used during the procedure; however, it is done on an out-patient basis. PEG feeding tubes are larger than naso-gastric feeding tubes so that crushed medication may go through it in addition to the tube feeding diet.*

✦ *A surgical gastrostomy feeding tube is also intended for long-term use by someone with no evidence of nausea and vomiting. It is inserted much like a PEG feeding tube;*

however it is done by a surgeon and while the patient is under general anesthesia. Oftentimes, it is inserted in conjunction with another surgical procedure.

✦ *A surgical jejunostomy feeding tube is used by people who require long-term feeding and have a history of chronic nausea and vomiting. It is sewn into the intestine by a surgeon while the patient is under general anesthesia. It is also usually done only if the person requires another surgical procedure.*

Formula Types and Administration

Over 100 products are available for use in a feeding tube. With your increased need for protein, we suggest selecting only "high-protein" or "high-nitrogen" diets. Usually, these contain over 18% of the total calories as protein.

SUSTACAL **HN**
   Manufacturer—Mead Johnson Nutritionals, Evansville, IN
800-247-7893 (nutrition and ordering information)

JEVITY
   Manufacturer—Ross Laboratories, Columbus, OH
800 227-5767 (nutrition information) or 800 544-7495 (order only)

ISOSOURCE **HN**
   Manufacturer—Sandoz Nutrition, Minneapolis, MN
800 999-9978

REPLETE
   Manufacturer—Clintec Nutrition, Deerfield, IL
800 422-2752 (nutrition information)

Each of the above formulas requires that you have a fully functioning intestine. If you have diarrhea or fat malabsorption, use any of the modified fat products (see page 82). All diets may be fed either into the stomach or into the intestine.

It is relatively simple to administer your own tube feeding diet. Most people prefer to receive the tube feeding formula while they sleep. It is safely administered at a slow constant rate with the help of a feeding pump, so you can eat what you like during the day without feeling full from the formula. People with a tube inserted in the stomach may use either a pump or a syringe, which allows for several ounces of the formula to be put in the stomach at a time. Usually dividing the daily formula amount into 4 to 6 doses is best; this mimics regular eating. All people with surgical jejunostomies need a pump and cannot have the formula administered in doses.

Intravenous Diets

An intravenous diet was first used in the early 1970s at the University of Pennsylvania to feed a young girl who was surely going to die of malnutrition because of a non-functioning gastrointestinal tract. A tube feeding formula would not have worked. An intravenous catheter was placed in the child's large vein that flows directly into the heart, and a nutritional solution was administered. The child did beautifully, and a new treatment of malnutrition was born—total parenteral nutrition (TPN).

TPN has been successful for thousands of people with a variety of health conditions, such as cancer, short bowel syndrome, Crohn's disease, and AIDS. Some of these conditions require TPN feeding for life; in other cases the TPN helps a person through a rough period when taking an oral diet or tube feeding formula is not possible. It is given to hospitalized patients who are too sick to eat, in an attempt to prevent malnutrition, but many others receive TPN at home.

Intravenous feeding is generally recommended for people with HIV infection when they have prolonged diarrhea, malabsorption of fat and other nutrients, anorexia that resists treatment by drugs, and a weight loss of over 10% of their usual weight. For HIV infection, TPN should not be viewed as a lifetime therapy. It can be used short-term, say for several months, to help you regain some weight and strength or administered several times a week to maintain a good weight and to avoid dehydration. TPN is most effective at restoring weight and a feeling of well-being when weight loss is around 10%.

If more weight is lost, it may not be as effective. In every case, though, it is mandatory that recipients of TPN are actively being treated for HIV infection; otherwise the TPN won't be effective.

The goal for using TPN is weight gain, both muscle and fat. If a secondary infection is present, it is likely that only fat will be gained. At those times, we encourage using TPN a little longer after the infection clears up so that some muscle can be restored. Of course, exercise, even mild forms such as walking, will build muscle. Most people gain 15 to 25 pounds with TPN but then seem to stop, even if they continue taking it. Nonetheless, a 20-pound weight gain or so is enough to improve appearance and increase strength.

There is some risk using TPN, especially because of the way in which it is given: into the major vein that leads directly to the heart. The needle inserted into this vein is exposed to air. Many physicians are reluctant to prescribe TPN for fear it will make the patient more prone to infections, but some published reports do not support this. People without HIV infection have used TPN at home for a couple of decades. Their immune system is compromised by cancer or bowel disease, but only less than 5% get serious infections related to the TPN. The statistics are the same for people with HIV infection.

If you seem to meet the criteria for TPN, it is important to discuss it with your doctor. Determine why TPN is or is not appropriate for you. If you disagree with your physician's advice, you may want to seek another opinion. Remember, it is quite possible to become very sick and have a worsening immune system from being too malnourished—and TPN treats malnutrition. You may want to bring up the subject of using TPN with your doctor—even if it's early in the course of the disease—to gain a better understanding of when its use is required. In addition, you may get a sense of your physician's feeling toward the therapy in general.

Types of Catheters

There are two ways in which the TPN can go into your vein. One is by a standard catheter such as a Hickman. This tubing is easy to hook up to the TPN solution. Because it is outside the skin and in contact with the open air, though, you need to be careful and cover it well, especially while wearing clothing and showering. The alternative, a "port," is placed under the skin. This is better for people who do not want to worry about covering up a catheter during showering or swimming. However, hooking up the TPN feeding means that a needle must be stuck into the port, which causes a little pain. Some people leave the needle in to avoid sticking themselves daily, but leaving it in too long increases the risk of infection. Be sure to review the pros and cons of each device with the surgeon who will place it.

A newer type of device can be placed into your arm by a nurse or a doctor in an out-patient setting. It is called a PICC line and is becoming more popular among our patients. It has a long line, which is threaded from your arm almost all the way to your heart. Our surgeons have found no difference in infection rates between the standard catheter and a port in patients with HIV infection.

Formulas and Administration

All TPN diets given are highly purified and sterile. They contain all of the macronutrients—carbohydrate, protein, fat, and water—in the amounts you would have been taking with an oral diet. They also contain micronutrients such as vitamins, minerals, and trace elements. If you have a lot of diarrhea and are losing electrolytes such as sodium and bicarbonate, the TPN allows you to replace these rapidly. In all, the TPN gives you macronutrients for weight gain and micronutrients to feel better.

TPN diets contain fat along with the other nutrients. Depending upon your needs, you will get fat either daily or several times a week; intravenous fat is efficiently stored, so it doesn't matter which. In any regard, you should gain only a pound a week, although you may gain more during the first couple of weeks because you are likely to be dehydrated at the start and are just filling up with water.

Most people receive the TPN while they sleep, over 10 to 12 hours. Some people are taking intravenous gancyclovir or foscarnet for CMV retinitis. In these cases, the TPN is administered overnight and the medication in the morning. Since the foscarnet requires that you receive extra fluids to avoid kidney damage, the TPN provides some of the extra fluid required.

Even if you are receiving TPN, you should try to eat during the day. It appears that the risk of infection is less when you eat conventional foods as well as take TPN. It doesn't have to be full meals; small amounts of a variety of foods that you crave are all right. As long as your intestine has to work to digest something periodically, it becomes stronger and better able to fight off infections.

Summary

With preventing malnutrition as your top goal, there may be a time when conventional foods are not enough. That's when you should turn to oral liquid supplements, tube feeding, or an intravenous diet. All three have been shown to promote weight gain in people with HIV infection. None are experimental. Tube feeding diets and TPN involve some risk, but with proper training, your risks are minimized.

Take the initiative in discussing the use of these different diets with your doctor. It's never too early. Even with the first 5 pounds of weight loss, you should schedule an appointment with your doctor to learn about your options.

meal planning & food preparation

by Maria Sachs

My grandmother cooked for us except on Sundays, when my father took over the kitchen. Unlike her careful, rather anxious productions, his were seemingly slapdash and never the same twice. He would poke around the 'fridge, pull out some meat, raw or cooked, and whatever else he fancied—sour cream, a tomato, garlic, Worcester sauce—then reach for the spices and start cooking. That rather casual approach to meals and food preparation forms the basis of this chapter.

Chances are that before you contracted HIV infection, you ate the same foods as everyone else. You had two main concerns: your health and your appearance. You would read in the newspaper and hear on TV and radio that fat, sugar, salt, and red meat were bad for you, while pasta and whole grains and fruit and vegetables were good for you. Milk was no longer a must, but if you did drink it, it was probably skimmed of fat.

You wanted to be healthy, and you wanted to look good—not too fat or too thin. You made tradeoffs: to eat some high-calorie foods you liked, you went without others. If you fancied some Häagen- Dazs one night after work, you may have had light soup and salad first so that you could eat a large bowl of ice cream without gaining weight.

And that was fine. It certainly did no harm to avoid the foods it was chic to avoid (red meat, saturated fat, dairy products, and so forth). Or to eat a light meal so that you could splurge on a non-nutritious high-calorie dessert. Now that has changed completely.

The eating habits that worked for you before HIV infection would now do just the opposite. You'd become tired and listless, you may lose weight, and your health may suffer. You'll have to cast aside all the old taboos. Red meat and milk are fine, in fact are needed. Sugar and salt won't hurt you, and as they enhance flavor, are especially useful during periods of anorexia. You can no longer skip meals or eat lightly to splurge on dessert. This is not to say that you can never eat high calorie, non-nutritious foods. Of course you can—but have them at the end of the day, after you've met your essential needs (see Chapter 2). Then, go ahead and have that sundae.

The upshot, of course, is that you need to eat according to the Principles of Positive Nutrition. Mainstream "healthy" American diets are unsuitable. You need a way to cook that will help you eat as you should without tedious measuring and calorie counting and without investing too much time or effort.

This chapter is devoted to simple meal planning and food preparation tips. It involves a few instructions and offers endless variety. There are no recipes (those come in Chapter 8), just a lot of combinations for you to try: various kinds of meat, cooked in different ways, with various ingredients and spices.

The nutrients you need daily are organized into tables of meat and fish plus three kinds of side dishes: starch, vegetables, and fruit desserts. As long as you get these in the right amounts, along with the required dairy products, you can add any soups, appetizers, desserts, or snacks you like. The tables show the name of the dish and the primary component—meat, rice, and so on—in capital letters in the first column; it then gives the other ingredients essential to the dish, in boldface where you need a quarter to half a cup or so, and in normal print where it's tablespoons or less. (That's quite a range, so adjust downward or upward as you see fit. And you'll want only teaspoons or less of some ingredients. With dried herbs, in particular, less is generally better). The second column lists optional ingredients, again in bold or normal print depending on amount, that you can add singly or in combination. Also noted are procedures for assembling your dish, any other comments, and also cooking method and time. At the start of most tables will be some general hints and comments.

To keep things as simple as possible, it's assumed that you know the rudiments of cooking, if not, consult a basic cookbook for tips. Salt and pepper are omitted throughout; just season to your taste. The dishes given take less than 15 minutes to prepare, and of course all meet the nutritional goals outlined earlier.

You can be relaxed about putting your dish together. Once you have the essential ingredient, you needn't weigh and measure the rest. Experiment a little: add your own favorites or swap them for others, and if you're missing some ingredient, use something else. After all, what can go wrong? Some dishes will just turn out better than others. After a while, you'll mix and match on you own, and will have vastly increased you repertoire.

Cooking Poultry, Beef, Pork, and Fish

All cooking reduces the uncooked weight of the meat, usually by about 10% to 20%. So if anything, buy a few more ounces than your protein needs require. More water is lost at higher temperatures and with longer cooking times, so baking meats at 350° could shrink them less than broiling for a long time at around 500°.

{cooking meats}

	CHICKEN	PORK	BEEF	FISH
Bake/Roast	325°	325° to 350°	300° to 350°	325°

to Sauté (pan fry)...

CHICKEN, DE-BONED CUTLET: Medium high, 3-4 minutes per side. Chicken should not be pink. Piercing with a fork should produce clear juice (not pink).

PORK, DE-BONED CUTLET: Medium high, 3-4 minutes per side: thicker pieces may need more time. Pork should never be pink; piercing with a fork should produce clear juice.

BEEF, DE-BONED: Medium high; time depends on thickness. Meat should be only a little pink

FISH: Medium high, 10 minutes per inch of thickness

Microwaving meat is not a good idea because it does not get cooked uniformly. This increases the risk of bacterial or microbial contamination in areas that are not cooked to a high enough temperature to kill all of these harmful organisms.

Poultry

A rule of thumb when you buy poultry is that 1/3 is bone and other inedible parts. This goes for chicken, turkey, and other poultry such as capon, duck, and goose. As Chapter 2 indicated, men need 100 to 120 grams of protein a day, while women need 80 to 100 grams. To figure out how much poultry to buy, you'll have to calculate the protein it contains. Let's say that of the 100 g of protein you need daily, you've consumed 40 grams by 4 p.m., and so you need another 60 grams. How much poultry do you buy for tonight's dinner? If it has bones and skin, you'll need:

60 g of protein = 9 ounces of meat (remember: all meats contain 7 g of protein per ounce, plus 2 ounces to allow for shrinkage)

11 ounces of edible poultry = x ounces of poultry with bones and skin

x = 3/2 x 11 ounces = 16.5 ounces

Of course, if you otherwise buy boneless, skinless poultry, just buy the 11 ounces.

Tips: Chicken likes rosemary, tarragon, and oregano. You may want to squeeze lemon juice over chicken about an hour before you start to cook. Fat-free yogurt seems to behave better when heated than yogurt containing fat. You can usually substitute sweet cream for sour cream. Garlic is always chopped or crushed, and always first glazed in 1/2 butter and 1/2 olive or canola oil.

For cooking wine, use dry vermouth so that you don't have to keep opening bottles. And don't cook with a wine you wouldn't drink. Many people prefer curry paste to powder. Buy your herbs at a health food store where they're fresher and much cheaper. And for less pungent garlic, take out the sprout down the center.

Poultry

ESSENTIAL INGREDIENTS	OPTIONAL INGREDIENTS

BAKED CHICKEN
- CHICKEN LEGS, THIGHS, or BREAST
- Equal parts condensed **mushroom or celery soup & sour cream or yogurt**
- sliced mushrooms or celery

✛ Mix and spread on chicken
✛ Bake at 350° for 1 hour

- lemon juice
- dry vermouth
- capers
- tarragon
- **bamboo shoots**

BAKED CHICKEN II
- CHICKEN LEGS, THIGHS, or BREAST
- **Sour cream or yogurt**

✛ Mix and spread over chicken
✛ Bake at 350° for 1 hour

- Worcestershire sauce
- lemon juice
- garlic
- bread crumb topping

PINK CHICKEN
- CHICKEN LEGS, THIGHS, or BREAST
- soy sauce
- Rose or red wine

✛ Brown chicken at medium heat in frying pan, then add everything else
✛ Bake uncovered at 350° for 1 hour

- garlic
- ginger root
- oregano
- sour cream
- **sliced mushrooms**

Bold text – use approximately 1/4 cup • Plain text – use approximately 1 Tbsp.

Poultry

| ESSENTIAL INGREDIENTS | OPTIONAL INGREDIENTS |

CURRIED CHICKEN (try also turkey, lamb, pork, or beef)

- CHUNKS OF COOKED MEAT
- curry paste
- **chopped onion**
- **yogurt**

- **tomato juice, bouillon, or water**
- chutney
- garlic
- chopped tomato, apple, or orange
- fresh chopped coriander

✤ Sauté onions and curry, then add everything except yogurt and meat

✤ Cook covered on medium heat 1/2 hour, then add yogurt and meat and heat thoroughly

TURKEY DIJON (try this also with pork)

- TURKEY BREAST or THIGH
- Equal parts **apricot jam** or allfruit & **Dijon mustard** (Also try peach jam or orange marmalade)

✤ Pour over turkey
✤ Bake uncovered 350° 1 hour

VIETNAMESE SALAD

- DICED COOKED CHICKEN or TURKEY
- blanched cabbage (white, savoy, or Chinese)
- crushed peanuts
- soy sauce

- oil
- lime juice
- a pinch of sugar
- scallions
- chopped fresh coriander
- garlic

✤ Mix and let stand for at least 1 hour in the refrigerator; eat at

Bold text – use approximately 1/4 cup • Plain text – use approximately 1 Tbsp.

Fish and Shellfish

Fish can be very simple to cook. It's amazing how little time it takes. Cook at 10 minutes per inch of height at 450° (and for 10 minutes if it less than an inch thick). Dense fish such as swordfish may take a little longer than flaky fish. If the fish is cooked in foil, it also needs longer. Test with a fork; the fish should not be clear or translucent inside—it must be thoroughly cooked. Fish likes lemon, mayonnaise, and white wine, bread crumbs, capers, and most herbs (used sparingly).

ESSENTIAL INGREDIENTS	OPTIONAL INGREDIENTS

MARIA'S SCALLOPS
- SCALLOPS
- melted butter

- garlic
- lemon
- thyme
- **bread crumb topping**

✦ Coat scallops in butter, then add the remaining ingredients
✦ Bake uncovered at 450°

BAKED FISH I
- SCROD, HADDOCK, or ANY FLAKY WHITE FISH

- mayonnaise
- lemon juice
- capers
- grated parmesan
- dill weed
- bread crumb topping

✦Spread mixture on fish
✦Bake uncovered 450°

Fish & Shellfish

ESSENTIAL INGREDIENTS	OPTIONAL INGREDIENTS
BAKED FISH II	
• BLUEFISH	• mustard
	• garlic
	• ginger
	• fresh chopped coriander
	• bread crumb topping
✤ Spread mixture on fish	
✤ Bake uncovered 450°	
SPECIAL SALMON	
• SALMON	• diced tomato & scallions
	• fresh parsley or
	• coriander
	• lemon juice
✤ Spread mixture on fish	
✤ Bake uncovered 450°	

Bold text – use approximately 1/4 cup • Plain text – use approximately 1 Tbsp.

Other meats

All meats must be thoroughly cooked. Again, onions are glazed first and garlic is chopped or crushed. All meats are browned in 1/2 canola oil and 1/2 butter before you add the rest of the ingredients. Beef tastes great with thyme and bay leaf; pork likes marjoram. And lamb is wonderful with cumin and coriander, and of course garlic.

ESSENTIAL INGREDIENTS	OPTIONAL INGREDIENTS

BEEF STROGANOFF

- CHUNKS or STRIPS OF BEEF
- * onions
- sour cream

- chopped dill pickle
- mustard
- sliced mushrooms

+ Brown meat, then add everything else
+ Cook on medium heat until meat is done (slightly pink inside)

BEEF GOULASH (or beef with pork or veal)

- CHUNKS OF MEAT
- onions
- sweet paprika

- beef stock (canned or cube)
- fruit juice or red wine
- diced pepper
- caraway seeds

+ Brown meat, then add the rest
+ Bake on medium-low heat covered 1-1/2 hours; add more liquids about every 20 minutes if needed

CURRIED BEEF OR LAMB (see curried chicken)

PORK DIJON

- PORK TENDERLOIN
- Equal parts **apricot or allfruit jam** & **Dijon mustard** (also try peach jam or orange marmalade)

+ Pour mixture over pork
+ Bake uncovered 350° 1 hour

Bold text – use approximately 1/4 cup • Plain text – use approximately 1 Tbsp.

Other Meats

ESSENTIAL INGREDIENTS	OPTIONAL INGREDIENTS

PORK CHOP CASSEROLE
- PORK CHOPS
- **concentrated tomato soup**

- chopped onions
- apple eighths
- sliced tomatoes
- thyme or marjoram

✛ Brown chops, add rest of ingredients
✛ Bake covered at medium-low heat 1 hour

MIDDLE-EASTERN LAMB
- COOKED LAMB CHUNKS (from roast or chops)
- yogurt
- **flour tortillas**

- chopped onions & scallions
- garlic
- cumin
- dried coriander

✛ Cook together, adding yogurt last, and heat thoroughly in frying pan
✛ Put on heated tortilla

BLUE LAMB CHOPS
- LAMB CHOPS
- Blue cheese

✛ Brown chops on one side, then turn & spread with blue cheese and cook until done (when meat is slightly pink)
✛ Pan fry

Starches

ESSENTIAL INGREDIENTS	OPTIONAL INGREDIENTS

RICE CASSEROLE
- COOKED RICE
- **sour cream**
- chopped red pepper

     • Jack cheese topping
     • cumin

+ Mix all ingredients
+ Bake at 350° for 30 minutes

WILD RICE SALAD
    Equal parts of:
- COOKED WILD RICE
(or 1/2 WILD and
1/2 WHITE),
- **chopped unsalted pecans,
and dried cranberries**
- grated orange rind
- orange juice

     • oil
     •chopped scallion
     •lemon juice

+ Mix and let stand for 30 minutes; eat at room temperature

POTATOES PROVENÇALES
- SMALL WHOLE
NEW POTATOES
- oil

     • **roughly chopped onion**
     • bay leaf
     • garlic
     • thyme

+ Toss potatoes in oil and add the rest
+ Bake covered 350° 45 minutes or longer

Bold text – use approximately 1/4 cup • Plain text – use approximately 1 Tbsp.

Starches

ESSENTIAL INGREDIENTS	OPTIONAL INGREDIENTS

SWEET POTATO BOATS
- SWEET POTATOES
- butter
- lemon
- vermouth

✛ Bake potatoes, cut lengthwise and scoop out, mix and refill skins

✛ Broil for a few minutes when refilled

JAZZY QUINOA

• COOKED QUINOA	• fresh chopped coriander
	• garlic
	• lemon juice

✛ Mix quinoa with other ingredients, let stand; eat at room temperature

TASTY PASTA

• COOKED PASTA	• parsley
•olive oil	• halved jalapeño peppers
• garlic	with seeds removed

✛ Heat garlic and peppers in oil; mix with hot pasta

GERMAN NOODLES
- COOKED EGG NOODLES
- equal parts sour
  cream & butter
- black pepper

✛ Mix everything with hot noodles

Bold text – use approximately 1/4 cup • Plain text – use approximately 1 Tbsp.

Vegetables

ESSENTIAL INGREDIENTS	OPTIONAL INGREDIENTS

LEEK AND PEPPERS SUPREME

• 1/2 inch-thick LEEK and RED PEPPER slices	• vinegar
• oil	• **cooked wild rice**
• soy sauce	• **torn-up lettuce**

✦ Sauté leek and peppers in oil, add soy sauce and rice or lettuce

✦ Heat thoroughly (until lettuce is wilted)

SUSAN'S ACORN SQUASH

• SQUASH, cut widthwise	• brown sugar
• oil or butter	• pecans
	• lemon juice

✦ Bake halves face down on oiled sheet; scoop out, discard seeds, mix and restuff

✦ First bake 45 minutes at 375°, then 5 minutes more after restuffing

GREEN BEAN CASSEROLE

• COOKED GREEN BEANS	• lemon juice
• Equal parts concentrated mushroom soup & sour cream or yogurt	
• bread crumb topping	

✦ Bake 350° for 45 minutes

Bold text – use approximately 1/4 cup • Plain text – use approximately 1 Tbsp.

Vegetables

ESSENTIAL INGREDIENTS	OPTIONAL INGREDIENTS

BROCCOLI WITH ALMONDS
- BROCCOLI FLOWERS
- almonds

- Equal parts **mayonnaise** & **sour cream or yogurt**
- grated parmesan
- chopped parsley

✚ Cook broccoli until crunchy; mix rest, warm, and spread over broccoli

BAKED CARROTS
- SMALL PEELED CARROTS
- butter

- **scallions**
- tarragon

✚ Wrap all tightly in foil
✚ Bake at 350° for 45 minutes or until soft

BUTTERNUT SQUASH
- PEELED DICED SQUASH
- butter

- brown sugar
- lemon juice
- pecans or almonds

✚ Purée cooked squash with other ingredients
✚ Steam squash

Bold text – use approximately 1/4 cup • Plain text – use approximately 1 Tbsp.

✚ 104 ✚

Fruits

ESSENTIAL INGREDIENTS	OPTIONAL INGREDIENTS

BAKED BANANAS
- BANANAS

- butter
- brown sugar
- lemon juice
- brandy

+ Slit skin of banana, add rest of ingredients except brandy; add brandy before serving
+ Bake at 300 °until soft

BAKED GRAPEFRUIT
- GRAPEFRUIT HALVES
- brown sugar
- brandy

+ Cut sections, add sugar; add brandy before serving
+ Bake at 300° until hot

SAUTÉED APPLES
- PEELED EIGHTHS OF GOLDEN DELICIOUS APPLES
- butter
- brown sugar

- lemon or orange rind
- lemon or orange juice
- brandy

+ Sauté 15 minutes or until soft
+ Add brandy before serving

Fruits

ESSENTIAL INGREDIENTS	OPTIONAL INGREDIENTS

BAKED PEARS
- UNPEELED TWELFTHS OF PEARS
- lemon juice
- brown sugar
- Grapenuts cereal
- butter

+ Top with grapenuts heated in butter
+ Bake uncovered at 350° for 30 minutes

Bold text – use approximately 1/4 cup • Plain text – use approximately 1 Tbsp.

+ 106 +

culturally diverse recipes

by Estelle Raiffa

For 14 years as a social worker in Boston, I counseled people living with HIV infection. Most of my clients recognized the importance of maintaining their weight and eating healthful foods. Those from other countries, however, had a strong desire to continue to eat their native foods and meals. At the same time, many of my clients were dealing with the demands of work, not feeling well, or at times not having the strength to cook. All of this prompted my interest in the problems associated with nutrition and cooking for people with HIV infection.

This chapter features the culturally diverse recipes I have collected over the years that are not only simple to prepare and delicious, but also are nutritionally adequate for anyone living with HIV infection. (The Positive Nutrition Pyramid food groups and number of servings that each recipe contains are included to help you plan your daily intake.) In addition, a number of recipes suggest "short-cuts" for those who don't feel well or are short on time. (It also helps to put all of the ingredients for a recipe on the kitchen counter before starting.) My hope is that no matter your ethnic background, if you enjoy cooking and trying new dishes, you'll enjoy these tasty dishes.

Leek and Potato Soup

From the kitchen of Estelle Raiffa

This is a delicious and basic soup to which you can add other vegetables, (watercress or broccoli), and additional cream or butter if you are trying to gain weight. My advice is to add cream to the individual plate, and not to the pot, since it will give you greater flexibility in reheating the leftovers.

4-5 Tablespoons of butter or margarine
4-5 large leeks, enough to make 6 cups, white and light
    green parts only, wash and cut across into thin slices
1 medium baking potato, peeled and diced
2 10.5-oz. cans condensed chicken broth
2 cans water (If you use uncondensed chicken broth, use 3
    14.5-oz. cans and omit water.)
salt, if needed

Heat butter in a soup pot over medium heat. Add leeks and stir for 5-10 minutes until leeks appear wilted. Add potato, chicken broth, and water to the leeks. Cover pot and simmer soup for about 30 minutes, until vegetables are soft. Put mixture, 2-3 cups at a time, through a blender. Add salt, if needed.

Serve hot or cold. A tablespoon of cream or a pinch of cumin added to the plate (not the pot) provides a different taste. If you divide this soup into two batches when you reheat it, you can add a bunch of washed and stemmed watercress and cook it with the soup for 10 minutes. Put the soup through the blender again and you have a new, different soup. You can do the same with 2-3 stalks of broccoli. Serves 6.

Positive Nutrition Exchanges: 2 fats & oils, 2 vegetables

Caldo Calego, a Mediterranean Soup

This is a Mediterranean soup offered by Ralph Bryant, Executive Chef at Rustica, a new Belmont, Massachusetts, restaurant; Bob Goodman is the proprietor.

1 Tablespoon light virgin olive oil or vegetable oil
1/2 lb. turkey, chicken or pork sausage
1 large onion, chopped (about 1 1/2 cups)
1 1/2 cups diced carrots
14.5-oz. can diced tomatoes
16-oz. can small white beans, rinsed and drained
3 medium potatoes, diced, (about 2 cups)
6 cups water
Salt and pepper to taste
1/4-1/3 package of frozen chopped spinach, defrosted and
    drained, or a few leaves of fresh spinach, cut up.

Brown sausage in Dutch oven or large pot, over medium heat, stirring often until browned. If sausage starts to stick to pot, add a little water. Cut sausage into bite-size pieces. Add onion and carrot, and mix with a large spoon. Cover and cook over a low heat until onion is softened, about 5 minutes. Add undrained tomatoes, beans, potatoes, water, salt, and pepper. Cover, and bring to a boil. Reduce heat, and simmer over low heat, covered, about 35 minutes. Uncover and simmer 10 minutes longer until vegetables are tender and soup is thickened. Stir in spinach and heat thoroughly.
    Serves 6.

Positive Nutrition Exchanges: 1 fat & oil, 2 vegetables, 1 grain & baked good

Bouillon with Egg, from Austria

This is a very simple soup that can be served for lunch, or as a first course at dinner. It is an Austrian soup that I enjoyed while living in Vienna.—Estelle Raiffa

10.5-oz. can beef broth
1 can water (If you prefer chicken broth, use 2 14.5-oz.
    uncondensed cans and omit water.)
2 eggs
2 teaspoons chives, cut up (optional)

Add water to broth and boil. Reduce heat to low, and simmer the soup. Gently drop in eggs into the soup, and cover the pot. Serve the soup when the eggs are poached and thoroughly cooked (about 5 minutes). Sprinkle chives over soup as a garnish (optional).
    Serves 2.

Positive Nutrition Exchanges: 1/3 high-protein food

Chinese Vegetable and Mushroom Soup

Contributed by Estelle Raiffa

4-6 black Chinese mushrooms
1 cup boiling water
2 Tablespoons of sesame oil
2-4 slices fresh ginger
1 small head bok choy, washed and cut across into thin
    slices
1 small head Chinese cabbage, washed and cut across into
    thin slices
2 10.5-oz. cans chicken broth
2 cans water
1 cooked chicken breast, cut into strips or bite-size pieces
6-8 snow peas
4 teaspoons tamari reduced-sodium soy sauce
1/2 teaspoon salt (more if needed)

Place mushrooms into one cup of boiling water and set aside for 30 minutes. Heat sesame oil, in a soup pot, over medium heat. Add ginger slices and sauté for 30 seconds

Add bok choy and Chinese cabbage, and stir until they appear wilted, about 5-10 minutes. Add chicken broth, 2 cans of water, the mushrooms, and the cup of water the mushrooms were steeped in. Add chicken strips. Cook over medium heat for 10-15 minutes. Add snow peas, and cook an additional 4-5 minutes. Add tamari and salt, to taste. Serve hot. Vegetables should be crunchy and not over-cooked.

Serves 4.

Positive Nutrition Exchanges: 1 fat & oil, 1 vegetable

Shrimp Seviche, a soup from Ecuador

This is a cold soup from Ecuador with a surprise ingredient. Faisal Baki contributed this recipe.

1 lb. medium shrimp, cooked and peeled,
    and cut in half lengthwise
1 cup freshly squeezed lemon juice
1 cup orange juice
1 cup ketchup
1 teaspoon hot sauce (Tabasco)
2 cups sliced onions
salt and pepper to taste
popcorn

Combine all of the ingredients. Add salt and pepper, to taste. Chill for 30 minutes. Serve with popcorn stirred into the soup.
    Serves 2.

Positive Nutrition Exchanges: 2 fruits, 2 vegetables, 2 high-protein foods

Mediterranean Fish Soup

Mike Moss is a musician who lives and works in Boston. He made this soup for our family one summer night. The recipe, really a one-dish meal, is from his mother Evelyn Moss.

1 pound can crushed tomatoes
1 large, or two medium size potatoes, cut into large chunks
1 green pepper, cut into strips
1 medium onion, cut up into small pieces
2 carrots, cut into chunks
2 stalks celery, cut into chunks
1 bay leaf
1/4 teaspoon oregano
1 tablespoon fresh parsley, cut up
1/2 teaspoon white sugar
1 clove garlic, crushed
salt and pepper, to taste
1 teaspoon zest (the grated skin of an orange)
1/4 teaspoon sweet Hungarian paprika
3/4 pound of scrod, cut up into large chunks
4-5 large, uncooked shrimp, shells removed

In a large soup pot, simmer all of the vegetables in the tomatoes and its liquid until the potatoes are soft, about 20 minutes. Add the orange zest and paprika, stir into the soup. Add the scrod and cook over low heat for 10-15 minutes (depending upon the size of the fish pieces). Add the shrimp and cook for an additional 5-6 minutes until the shrimp are thoroughly cooked and look red. Garnish each soup bowl with a little extra fresh parsley, cut up (optional). Serve with crusty French or sour dough bread. Serves 3.

**Positive Nutrition Exchanges: 2 vegetables,
  1 high-protein food**

Sweet and Sour Cabbage Soup, Russian Style

From the kitchen of Estelle Raiffa

This soup reheats very well and tastes even better the next day. Do not put sour cream into the soup pot, as it will curdle in the reheating.

1 teaspoon vegetable oil
1-2 pounds beef shank, center cut, bone in
1 large onion, sliced
1 1/2 cups water
1/2 small cabbage, shredded, or half a bag of packaged
    coleslaw
16 oz. sauerkraut
1 large can stewed or crushed tomatoes
4-6 Tablespoons brown sugar
1/2 cup light golden raisins (optional)
1 teaspoon salt
1 Tablespoon sour cream, per plate (optional)

Heat oil over medium heat in a soup pot. Sear bones or meat in oil, and remove temporarily from the pot. Add onion and water to the pot and cook until water boils.

Return meat or bones to the pot, and add all remaining ingredients. Simmer on top of stove for two hours. Adjust sugar and salt seasoning, to taste. The soup should have a sweet and sour flavor.

Serve hot, with a marrow bone or a piece of the meat in the individual plate. Add a dollop of sour cream to the plate, if desired.

Serves 6.

Positive Nutrition Exchanges: 1 fat & oil, 2 vegetables, 1/2 high-protein food

Caribbean Chicken and Squash Stew

This delicious recipe is from Executive Chef Dannie Kelly of Community Servings, a federally funded daily meals program that feeds housebound AIDS patients in their Boston homes.

3-lb. broiler-fryer chicken, cut into 8 pieces
2 Tablespoons vegetable oil
2 medium onions, sliced
1/2-1 teaspoon crushed red pepper (add more if you like it very hot)
1/2 teaspoon leaf thyme, crumbled
1 cup chicken broth
16-oz. can stewed tomatoes
1 teaspoon salt
1 lb. smoked pork butt cut into 1/2 inch cubes
1/4 cup shredded coconut
2 large sweet potatoes, cut into chunks
1 medium size butternut squash, cut into chunks
10-oz. package frozen green peas

Brown chicken, a few pieces at a time, in oil in a large Dutch oven or heavy pot. Remove chicken pieces as they brown and set the aside. Add onions to drippings and sauté until golden in color. Stir in crushed red pepper and thyme.

Return chicken to pot. Add chicken broth, stewed tomatoes, salt, pork, and coconut and bring to boil.

Lower heat, cover pot, and simmer for 15 minutes. Add sweet potatoes and squash, and simmer 35-40 minutes or until chicken and vegetables are tender. Stir in green peas in the last 5 minutes. Serve with rice or crunchy bread. Serves 4.

Positive Nutrition Exchanges: 3 fats & oils, 1 vegetable, 1 grain & baked good, 2 high-protein foods

Tuna with Chick peas, Sri Lanka-style

This is a light luncheon dish, contributed by Suki Devarajin, a graduate student in the Mason Fellows Program at Harvard.

6-oz. can tuna fish, drained
1 cup chick peas, drained from the can
1 small tomato, cut up into small pieces
juice of 1 lime
salt and pepper to taste

Combine all ingredients. Chill and serve. Serves 2.

For another variation, add 1/4 teaspoon of cumin powder to the soup.

Positive Nutrition Exchanges: 2 high-protein foods

Tuscan Tuna and Bean Salad

This recipe was contributed by Joan Levitt, an excellent and imaginative cook who lives in Belmont, Massachusetts.

1/4 cup olive oil
1 1/2 Tablespoons red wine vinegar
Lots of freshly ground pepper, to taste
12-oz. can Cannellini beans, drained and rinsed
12-oz. can tuna in water, drained
1/2 red onion, chopped (approx. 1/3 cup)
2 Tablespoons parsley, chopped

Whisk first three ingredients together in a bowl. Add remaining ingredients to this vinaigrette. Prepare at least one hour before serving.
Serves 4.

Positive Nutrition Exchanges: 1 fat & oil, 1 grain & baked good, 1 high-protein food

Chicken with Leeks and Ginger

A variation of chicken with Japanese-style sauce

Half a chicken, cut into eighths (As with any chicken
  recipe, you can substitute all dark or all light chicken
  as you prefer.)
1 teaspoon salt
2 tablespoons canola or light virgin olive oil
2 cups of leeks, white and light green parts only, washed
  and cup into small pieces
1 1/2 cups small carrots or carrot chunks
3-4 slices of fresh ginger
1/4 cup of tamari sauce or soy sauce with reduced sodium
3/4 tablespoon brown sugar

Wash and dry chicken with paper towel and sprinkle salt over the pieces. Heat the oil in a pot over medium high heat. Add the chicken and brown lightly in the oil for about 5-6 minutes and set aside on a plate.

Add the leeks to the oil and sauté on medium heat until leeks are wilted, about 6-7 minutes. Add the ginger slices and the carrots to the leeks, and saute together for another 3-4 minutes, stirring frequently. Add the Tamari sauce to the brown sugar and pour it into the leeks-carrot-ginger mixture. Stir together. Add the chicken to the pot, and stir together.

Cover the pot, reduce the heat to low, and simmer the chicken for 30-35 minutes. If there isn't enough gravy, add a little cold water to the pot, and stir it into the mixture. Serve with flat noodles or rice. Serves 2.

Positive Nutrition Exchanges: 3 fats & oils, 3 vegetables, 2 high-protein foods

Curried Lima Beans and Chicken Wings

This is another delicious recipe from Chef Dannie Kelly of Community Servings in Boston.

3/4 lb. dried lima beans
4 cups water
1/4 cup butter or margarine
8 chicken wings, drum sticks or thighs, in any
    combination
1 large onion, chopped
6 carrots, sliced
2 teaspoons curry powder
1/4 teaspoon ground cinnamon
2 Tablespoons flour
2-3 teaspoons salt
10-oz. package frozen green peas

Cover beans with 4 cups of water and bring to boil for two minutes. Remove from heat and let stand, covered, for one hour. Melt butter in a large skillet. Add chicken and cook slowly until brown. Remove the chicken. Add onion, carrots, curry powder, and cinnamon to fat remaining in skillet. Sauté until onion is tender. Stir in flour and salt.

Drain beans, reserving liquid. If there are not two cups of liquid, add water. Add the liquid to the flour mixture. Cook, stirring constantly, until thickened. Bring to boil. Combine beans, chicken, and curry sauce in a 3- to 4-quart baking dish. Cover and bake at 350° for 30 minutes or until beans are tender, stirring once.

Boil frozen peas in 1/2 cup salted water for 3 minutes. Sprinkle them over the chicken just before serving. This dish reheats well, and makes wonderful leftovers the next day. Serves 4.

Positive Nutrition Exchanges: 1 fat & oil, 2 vegetables, 1 high-protein food

Italian Baked Stuffed Breast of Chicken

This recipe is from Bob Hornstein a chef and friend of author Stacey Bell.

1 whole boneless breast of chicken(6 ounces)
salt and freshly ground pepper, to taste
Fontina cheese, sliced thinly
4 asparagus spears (with ends trimmed), or cut thicker
    asparagus in half lengthwise
1/4 cup Italian-seasoned bread crumbs
1 teaspoon olive oil

Preheat oven to 350°. Place chicken breast between 2 sheets of wax paper. Pound chicken to an even thickness. Sprinkle chicken with salt and pepper. Flip over and salt and pepper the other side. On one half of breast place a slice of Fontina cheese and 4 asparagus spears. Place second slice of fontina cheese over the asparagus. Fold other half of breast over like a book. Sprinkle light coating of Italian-seasoned bread crumbs over each side of chicken breast. Place in baking dish, and drizzle olive oil over the top.

Bake for approximately 30 minutes. Chicken is done when springy to the touch.

Serves 1.

**Positive Nutrition Exchanges: 1 fat & oil, 1 vegetable,
1 grain & baked good, 2 high-protein foods**

Chicken Piccata

This is another recipe from Bob Hornstein, who says it is a "twist on a classic Italian dish."

2 boneless breasts of chicken (6 ounces each)
1/4 cup flour, seasoned with salt and pepper to taste
2 Tablespoons butter
1 cup sliced mushrooms
1 small can artichoke hearts, drained and sliced
1/4 cup dry vermouth
1/3 cup chicken broth
Lemon slices

Place chicken between 2 sheets of waxed paper. Pound the chicken for even thickness. Cut the chicken into bitesized pieces, and dredge in the seasoned flour, shaking off the excess.

Melt butter in a heavy large skillet over medium-high heat. Place chicken in skillet, do not crowd pieces, and sauté for approximately 5 minutes per side. Chicken should be browned but not cooked all the way through. When you turn the chicken, add mushrooms and artichoke hearts. Cook chicken on second side for about 4-5 minutes.

Add vermouth and chicken broth. Bring liquid to a boil and immediately reduce heat to simmer. Cover and cook for 15-20 minutes. Liquid should become syrupy but not too thick.

Serve over white rice, garnished with thin slices of lemon.

Serves 2.

Positive Nutrition Exchanges: 3 fats & oils, 2 vegetables, 2 high-protein foods

Poulet Foley

This elegant French dish is easy to make and comes from Peg Foley. It is from the Greenhouse Cookbook.

3 lb. frying chicken cut up
1/2-1 teaspoon salt
3 oz. sweet butter (or 2 Tablespoons butter and
    1 Tablespoon oil)
1 cup mushrooms, sliced
3 oz. brandy
1/2-1 cup heavy sweet cream
3 Tablespoons sherry

Wash and dry the chicken; sprinkle with salt. Melt butter; add chicken, and brown on all sides. Cook, covered, over low heat, for 25-30 minutes, basting frequently with the butter. Add mushrooms, and sauté for three minutes. Pour brandy over chicken and mushrooms, ignite and let it burn for a few seconds. Add cream and sherry, and cook over low heat another 10 minutes.
    Serves 4.

Positive Nutrition Exchanges: 3 fats & oils, 2 high-protein foods

Baked Chicken, Greek Style

This recipe comes from the Greenhouse Cookbook.
Anne S. Antony contributed the recipe.

One-half frying chicken, cut in quarters (3 lbs. whole
    chicken)
Salt and pepper, to taste
Juice of 1/2 lemon
1/4 teaspoon oregano
1 teaspoon butter
1 teaspoon olive oil
1/2 cup boiling water

Preheat oven to 375°. Wash and dry chicken; season with salt and
pepper. Rub lemon juice and oregano into the chicken.

Put butter, oil, and water into pot. Add chicken. Bake, covered,
for 1 hour; baste after 30 minutes.

Serve with rice. Serves 2.

**Positive Nutrition Exchanges: 1 fat & oil, 2 high-protein
    foods**

Balsamic Spiked Chicken, French style

Bob Hornstein says, "This French-influenced dish is easy to prepare and makes a beautiful presentation." I agree!

1 whole roasting chicken (3-5 lb.)
2 large finely diced shallots
1/3 cup balsamic vinegar
1/3 cup Dijon mustard

Preheat oven to 350°. Wash and dry the chicken, remove the fat, and clean thoroughly. Slide your fingers underneath the skin and separate it from the chicken, but leaving it intact. In a small bowl combine shallots, vinegar, and mustard. Spoon the mixture under the skin of the chicken, pushing mixture throughout entire chicken. Also use marinade to coat the outside of the chicken. (A smaller chicken won't need as much marinade, and the quantities can be reduced by half.)

Place chicken in roasting pan, uncovered, and bake. Cooking time will vary based on the weight of the chicken. Figure 15-20 minutes per pound. The outside of the chicken should be well browned. Chicken is done when thigh is pierced with a fork and the juices run clear.

Remove the chicken from the oven and set aside, lightly covered with foil, for 10 minutes. Remove chicken from the pan and degrease pan juices. Carve and serve chicken, pouring a small amount of pan juices over the top.

Serves 4.

Positive Nutrition Exchanges: 2 high-protein foods

Chicken à La Creole

This recipe was contributed by Marie-Rose Romain Murphy, who was born and raised in Haiti, where she says she "learned to enjoy hot and spicy food." Mrs. Murphy is the Main Streets Program Director in Dorchester, Massachusetts.

1/4 cup canola oil
3 Tablespoons crushed garlic (3-4 cloves) or 2 teaspoons
    garlic powder
1 Tablespoon tomato paste
1 small cut-up chicken (about 3 lbs.)
1 large sliced onion
1 cup fresh parsley, chopped or 2 Tablespoons dry parsley
1/4 cup grated Romano cheese
3/4 jar (1 cup) Soffrito (a Goya sauce)
1/4 cup lemon juice
1/3 cup soy sauce
1/4-1/2 teaspoon Tabasco or Louisiana Hot Sauce, to taste

Mix the oil, garlic, and tomato paste and heat over a high flame. Sauté the chicken parts in this mixture until the chicken is brown. Add the onions and parsley, and stir the mixture until the onions are softened. Add the remaining ingredients. Reduce the temperature to medium-low heat and simmer until the chicken is cooked (30-40 minutes, depending upon the amount of chicken).

Serve with rice and Goya Black Bean Soup as a complementary sauce for the rice, suggests Mrs. Romain Murphy.

Serves 4.

Positive Nutrition Exchanges: 2 fats & oils, 2 high-protein foods

Piquant Turkey Breast

I make this for company, and use leftovers for turkey salad.

1 small frozen turkey breast, about 4 pounds
1/2-1 teaspoon salt
3 leeks, use white and pale green parts only
2 Tablespoons butter or canola oil
3 carrots, cut in large pieces
1/2 cup Dijon mustard
1/2 cup apricot preserves
1/2 cup chicken broth

Preheat oven to 325°. Thaw the turkey breast according to directions. Wash turkey and dry with paper towels. Sprinkle salt inside and outside the turkey, about 1/2-1 teaspoon, to taste. Set the turkey aside.

Sauté the leeks in butter or oil, on medium heat, until they look wilted, about 5 minutes. Add the carrots and sauté for 2-3 minutes. Place the sautéed vegetables in a baking dish. Place the turkey on the vegetables.

Mix the Dijon mustard and apricot preserves together and spread over the outside of the turkey breast. Do this while the turkey is in the pan so that any drippings remain in the pan. Roast the turkey, uncovered, in oven for 20 minutes per pound. (A 4-pound turkey should take about 80 minutes.) When the turkey is half cooked, add chicken broth to the pan gravy. Baste the turkey once or twice with the gravy. When the turkey is cooked, remove it from the oven and let rest in the pan for 15-20 minutes; this keeps the juices inside the turkey meat. Slice the turkey. Pour reheated gravy over the slices and serve with rice. Refrigerate leftover turkey immediately. Serves 6.

Positive Nutrition Exchanges: 1 fat & oil, 2 high-protein foods

Turkey Salad, from leftovers

1/2-3/4 cup mayonnaise (Do not use low-fat mayonnaise.)
1 Tablespoon tomato ketchup
1 teaspoon curry powder
4 cups cold turkey, cut up
2 stalks celery, chopped, approximately 1/2 cup
2 scallions or red onion, chopped (1/3 cup)
1/3 cup drained pineapple chunks

Mix together mayonnaise, ketchup, and curry powder. Add remaining ingredients and mix. Refrigerate 1-2 hours. Serve with lettuce and sliced tomatoes. Sprinkle slivered almonds or pecans over the top of the salad.

Serves 4.

Positive Nutrition Exchanges: 3 fats & oils, 2 high-protein foods

Shrimp Scampi

This is an Italian dish that is very quick to make and is very delicious. My husband and I like a lot of garlic in this dish, and while I've suggested quantities of garlic to use, you will want to add more or less according to your own taste.

6-8 medium size fresh (not frozen) shrimp, uncooked,
 with shells on
4-8 cloves of garlic, more or less to taste
2 Tablespoons of light virgin olive oil or canola oil
salt to taste (approximately 1/4-1/2 teaspoon, depending
 on amount of shrimp)

Remove shells from uncooked shrimp, divide shrimp by cutting a line down the back of the shrimp and pulling out the black "line." (This is easy to do but is actually optional.) Set the shrimp aside. Remove papery skin from garlic cloves and slice the clove in half, lengthwise. In a frying pan over low heat, sauté garlic in olive oil. When the garlic has turned a pale yellow color, turn heat to high and add shrimp. Cook shrimp for 5-6 minutes, until shrimp are red and cooked. Sprinkle salt over the shrimp as you stir them in the pan.

Serve the shrimp with the garlic oil in a soup bowl. Serve crusty French or Italian bread for dipping into sauce. Serves 1.

Optional variations:
  + add 1/4 cup white wine toward the end of cooking
  + lemon juice over shrimp at the end of cooking and sprinkle chopped parsley over shrimp

Positive Nutrition Exchanges: 6 fats & oils, 2 high-protein foods

Chinese Steamed Fish

Ying He, called "Heather," was born and raised in Beijing, China, where she studied art. Since emigrating to the U.S. ten years ago, she has become a successful artist. I met Ying He when she came to dinner with her fiancé, my nephew .

1 whole fresh fish, eviscerated, or two filets of fish (not frozen). Can use bass or red snapper or any small fresh fish.
salt and pepper, to taste
2-3 whole green scallions cut in half
6-7 thin slices of fresh ginger
2-3 Tablespoons of soy sauce
2-3 Tablespoons hot oil (canola oil or sesame oil, or a combination)

Use a wok or any pan with a cover that will steam fish. The fish should steam on a plate over a grill in the pan that keeps the fish away from the boiling water.

Wash and dry the fish and sprinkle it with salt and pepper to taste. Put the fish on a plate. Put scallions and three slices of ginger inside the fish, or between the two halves. Sprinkle soy sauce over the top of the fish, and place the remaining slices of ginger on top of the fish. Steam the fish for 7-8 minutes, depending upon its thickness. The pan should be tightly covered for proper steaming.

After the fish is cooked, remove it from the steamer, keeping it on the plate. Remove the ginger and scallions from the middle of the fish. Pour the very hot oil over the fish, and add more soy sauce, if needed. Discard the ginger, but use the scallions as a vegetable.

Serves 2-4, depending upon the size of the fish.

Positive Nutrition Exchanges: 2 fats & oils, 2 high-protein foods

Grilled Swordfish

*This is a summertime favorite of Bob Hornstein. He says
this dish can be rounded out with skewered vegetables and
apple pie for dessert.*

Fresh swordfish steaks, 6-8 oz. each, one steak per person
Salt
Ground white pepper
Mayonnaise (Do not use low-fat mayonnaise.)
Paprika
Lemon wedges

Wash and dry fish. Sprinkle each steak with salt and freshly ground
pepper (white pepper if you have it). Spread one side of each steak
with a "healthy amount" of mayonnaise, covering completely.
Sprinkle with paprika. Place mayo side down on heated grill. While
first side is grilling, spread top side of each steak with additional
mayonnaise. Cooking time will vary based on thickness of steaks
and level of heat from the grill. Be careful not to overcook. Serve
fish with wedges of lemon.

**Positive Nutrition Exchanges: 1 fat & oil, 2 high-protein
    foods**

Mayonnaise Fish

1/2 lb. fish per person of either haddock, scrod, cod or
salmon
Salt and pepper
Mayonnaise (Do not use low-fat mayonnaise.)
Sweet Hungarian paprika
Lemon juice
Lemon wedges

Wash and dry the fish. Sprinkle with salt and pepper, to taste.
Spread mayonnaise over one side of fish, sprinkle with paprika and
lemon juice. Place fish on broiling pan, and broil about 8 inches
from oven broiler. When mayonnaise on fish turns medium brown,
turn off broiler and bake fish, uncovered, in 325° oven for 25-30
minutes, depending on the thickness of the fish. Serve with lemon
wedge. Note: This fish goes well with small broiled red potatoes
and a steamed or stir-fried green vegetable.

Positive Nutrition Exchanges: 1 fat & oil, 2 high-protein foods

Medallions of Pork in Mustard Cream Sauce

Bob Hornstein, a chef and friend of Stacey Bell, says "this French-inspired dish is a wonderful special occasion meal because of the very high fat content, but it is also good for an everyday dinner because it's easy to prepare." Match this dish with rice pilaf and some steamed carrots and green beans for a colorful plate.

1 1/2 lb. pork tenderloin (Make sure as much of the fat as possible is removed.)
1/4 cup flour, seasoned with salt and pepper to taste
3-4 Tablespoons butter
3-4 scallions, white and pale green parts only (use green parts for garnish)
1/3 cup dry white wine
1/2 cup whipping cream
3 Tablespoons Dijon mustard

Slice pork into 3/4 inch thick slices. Place meat between 2 pieces of wax paper and pound to flatten the meat. Dredge the meat in flour that has been seasoned with salt and pepper. Melt 2 Tablespoons butter in large sauté pan over medium-high heat. Add meat and cook in batches about 4 minutes per side. As meat finishes cooking, place meat on plate and cover with foil. Add additional butter to sauté pan, as needed.

When all meat is cooked, add scallions, white and pale green parts only, to same skillet with an additional tablespoon of butter. Sauté over medium heat for 2 minutes.

Add wine to pan and bring to a boil. Reduce heat and cook, shaking pan frequently, until almost all liquid evaporates. Pour whipping cream into pan and return heat to high. Stir in mustard. Stir constantly over medium-high heat until sauce thickens, adjusting heat if boiling becomes too rapid. Taste sauce and adjust salt and pepper to taste. Place pork medallions on plate (3 slices per person) and spoon sauce over and around the pork. Garnish with green parts of scallions. Serves 4.

PLEASE NOTE: reduce the amount of the butter, wine, cream, scallions and mustard with a smaller piece of meat.

Positive Nutrition Exchanges: 3 fats & oils, 2 high-protein foods

Veal and Noodles With Sour Cream, Hungarian Style

This recipe by Kay Peckham comes from the Greenhouse Cookbook, *which was published by the Columbia University Greenhouse Nursery School in 1956.*

2 Tablespoons butter, divided
1 lb. stewing veal, cut in 1 inch cubes
3/4 teaspoon salt
1/2 teaspoon thyme
1 bay leaf
1 cup water
1/4 lb. mushrooms, peeled and sliced
4 oz. wide noodles
1/2 cup sour cream
1 oz. dry vermouth

Preheat oven to 350°. Melt 1 tablespoon butter in a casserole. Brown the veal with the seasonings (salt, thyme, bay leaf) in the butter. After meat is browned, add water, cover, and simmer one hour.

Brown mushrooms in remaining 1 tablespoon butter. Add to the veal during the last 15 minutes of cooking. Cook noodles according to package directions, drain and mix into veal. Stir in sour cream and vermouth. Bake in covered casserole for 20 minutes.

Serves 4.

Positive Nutrition Exchanges: 2 fats & oils, 1 grain & baked good, 1 high-protein food

Stir Fried Beef, Indonesian Style

This recipe was submitted by Carol Grodzins, Director of the Mason Fellows program at Harvard University.

1 lb. sirloin tips or rump steak
1 medium onion, quartered
5-10 whole peppercorns (optional)
1-3 garlic cloves, to taste
1/4 cup soy sauce
1/4 cup brown sugar
pinch of nutmeg
1 onion, sliced and set aside
2 Tablespoons of oil (olive or canola)
2 Tablespoons tomato paste or chopped fresh tomato

Slice the beef into thin slices. Combine onion, peppercorns, garlic, soy sauce, brown sugar, and nutmeg in a blender, and mix together. Marinate the sliced meat in the sauce for one to three hours in the refrigerator.

When ready to stir-fry, sauté sliced onion in oil, on high heat for 2-3 minutes. Add the meat and marinade to the onion; stir. Add the tomato paste or chopped tomato (the tomato paste makes a richer sauce). Turn the heat down to medium and stir until meat is tender (about 10-15 minutes).

Serve over rice. Serves 2

Positive Nutrition Exchanges: 3 fats & oils, 1 vegetable, 2 high-protein foods

Pastelon, a Puerto Rican recipe

*This dish was contributed by James Figueroa and his
mother who was born and raised in Puerto Rico.*

4 yellow (ripe*) plantains
1 lb. ground beef
1 Tablespoon butter
1 medium size green or red bell pepper, chopped
1 small onion (optional), chopped
1 packet of Goya Sazon seasoning
1/2 teaspoon oregano
1-3 crushed garlic cloves, or 1 teaspoon garlic powder
2-3 teaspoons Goya Adobo powder
4-6 shakes of Tabasco sauce
1 1/2 cups grated cheddar cheese

Peel the plantains, place in water to cover, and boil for 20-40 minutes, until they are soft. Remove the plantains from the water, slice
them, lengthwise into 3 strips and set them aside. Brown ground
beef in butter (15-20 minutes); drain and discard excess fat from the
pan. Add the onion, green pepper, and all of the seasonings.

Stir fry everything together until the meat appears "dry." Butter
a small baking pan (such as a lasagna pan), and layer the ingredients in this order:

strips of sliced plantain,
1/3 of the cheddar cheese
all of the meat mixture
1/3 of the cheese
strips of sliced plantain
1/3 of the cheese

Cover the baking pan with aluminum foil, and bake at 350° for 30-40 minutes. Remove from oven, let it rest for 10 minutes, then serve with rice. Serves 4.

* To ripen a plantain, leave it out for six to eight days. The skins will turn black when the fruit is ripe.

Positive Nutrition Exchanges: 1 dairy food, 1 fat & oil, 1 fruit, 1 high-protein food

Pigeon Pea Pelau

This recipe was given to me by Gloria Buffonge, a secretary at the Harvard Business School. Ms. Buffonge is from Virgin Gorda, the British Virgin Islands.

"This recipe can be made with any type of meat or chicken. Curry powder can also be added if you want it more spicy, and to give the dish a different flavor," she says.

1 Tablespoon canola or olive oil
1 1/2 lb. chicken (quarters), or 1 lb. beef (cubed)
1 large onion, chopped
1 small green pepper, chopped
1 large tomato, peeled and chopped
1 clove garlic, chopped
1/4 teaspoon thyme
1/4 teaspoon dried parsley (or use 2 teaspoons fresh
     parsley)
1/2 teaspoon salt, to taste
     4 cups water or chicken stock
1-1/2 cups uncooked rice
15-oz. can Goya pigeon peas, rinsed and drained

Heat oil and brown the chicken 15 minutes in a heavy pot, stirring occasionally to prevent sticking. (Brown beef for 5 minutes.) Add onion, and sauté until it turns pale yellow. Add the green pepper, tomato, and seasonings, and cook together about 5 minutes. Add water or chicken stock, rice, and pigeon peas, and bring to a boil.

Stir all ingredients, and lower the heat, and cover the pot and continue cooking until all liquid is absorbed and the rice is tender (about 35 minutes). Serves 4.

Positive Nutrition Exchanges: 1 fat & oil, 1 vegetable, 2 grains & baked goods, 1 high-protein food

Kourma Challow

This recipe was contributed by Helmand, a fine Afghanistan restaurant in Cambridge, Massachusetts. Challow is the rich accompaniment to the dish (see following recipe).

1/2-3/4 cup canola oil
2 large onions, chopped
2- to 2-1/2-lb. leg of lamb, boneless, cut into
    2 oz. pieces
2 large tomatoes, peeled and chopped
1 teaspoon salt, use more or less to taste
1/4-1/2 teaspoon black pepper, use more or less to taste
1-2 cloves fresh garlic, chopped
2-3 teaspoons coriander powder, adjust to taste
1/2-1 teaspoon turmeric powder, adjust to taste
1-1/2-2 cups water
2 large potatoes, peeled and cut into six pieces
1/4-1/2 lb. fresh green beans, these may be cut lengthwise
    in half
1 small cauliflower (just the flowers, not the stem)
1/8 lb. sun-dried tomatoes

Sauté onions in oil over medium heat until onions turn yellow. Add meat, raise heat to high, and sauté for 5 minutes until meat is thoroughly browned. Add tomatoes, and stir for 5 minutes more. Reduce heat to medium, and add salt, pepper, garlic, coriander, turmeric, and water. Stir all together quickly, cover pan, and simmer for one hour. Add the potatoes, and cook for 5 minutes, covered. Add the string beans, and cook for 5 minutes, covered. Add the cauliflower and sun-dried tomatoes and cook another 10-15 minutes, covered. Serve with Challow rice. Serves 4

Positive Nutrition Exchanges: 3 fats & oils, 2 vegetables, 2 high-protein foods

Challow Rice

3 cups basmati rice
1/2 teaspoon salt
1/2 cup canola oil
1 cup water, boiled
1/2 Tablespoon cumin powder

Wash and soak the rice in water to cover one hour prior to cooking
Preheat oven to 350°.

Fill a large cooking pot with 1 cup fresh water and bring it to a
boil. Add the rice, and boil for 5 minutes. Drain the rice in a colan-
der. Pour the rice into an oven-safe pot. Add salt, oil, water, and
cumin powder. Mix well.

Make the rice into the shape of a pyramid or hill. Make 5- or
6- inch holes in the rice with the end of a spatula. Cover the pot and
bake for one hour.

Serve with the Kourma. Serves 4.

**Positive Nutrition Exchanges: 2 fats & oils, 2 grains & baked
goods**

Cambodian Island Fried Rice with Chicken and Shrimp

This delicious recipe was contributed by Ann Berliner, a former teacher of learning-disabled children, who lives in Lexington, Massachusetts.

2 medium onions, chopped
2 medium green peppers, chopped
2-4 Tablespoons bacon fat
2 cups of cold, cooked rice (you can use one cup of white rice and one cup of brown rice)
1 teaspoon paprika (hot)
2 teaspoons celery salt, or one finely chopped fresh long celery stalk
1 teaspoon allspice
1 teaspoon fresh ginger, finely grated
2 Tablespoons brown sugar
4-6 Tablespoons soy sauce (low sodium), to taste
2 cups of cooked shrimp or chicken (or use one cup of each). Don't overcook shrimp or chicken since they will bake in the oven. But, be sure there is no red left in the chicken and that the shrimp can be cut with a fork easily.
1 pound baked ham, cut into small pieces, or use 1/4 pound of cooked bacon, instead
1 can (large) pineapple chunks, drained

Preheat oven to 350°.

Sauté onions and green pepper in 1-2 tablespoons of bacon fat. Remove onions and green pepper from the pan to a plate. Add more bacon fat, as needed (1 tablespoon) and stir-fry rice for 1-2 minutes in the fat. Add paprika, celery salt, allspice, ginger, brown sugar, and soy sauce. Add the cooked onions and green pepper and remove mixture from the heat. Add shrimp or chicken, ham, and

Cambodian Island Fried Rice with Chicken and Shrimp, continued

pineapple chunks to the mixture. Place mixture into lightly greased casserole, garnish with some extra pineapple chunks, and bake for 30 minutes. Serve with bread and salad. Serves 4.

Positive Nutrition Exchanges: 1 fat & oil, 1 fruit, 1 vegetable, 1 grain & baked good, 2 high-protein foods

Spicy Beef and Beans Stew

This recipe was contributed by Marie-Rose Romain Murphy, who was born and raised in Haiti, and who now lives and works in Massachusetts.

1 lb. steak tips, cut into bite-size chunks
2 Tablespoons olive oil
3 teaspoons garlic powder or 4-5 fresh cloves, crushed
2 Tablespoons dry parsley, or 4 Tablespoons fresh parsley, chopped
1 small onion, chopped
4 plum tomatoes, chopped or sliced
1 can Goya red kidney beans, drained and washed
1/4 cup red wine
2 1/2 Tablespoons balsamic vinegar
1/3 cup soy sauce
3 Tablespoons spaghetti sauce or tomato sauce
1/4-1/2 teaspoon Tabasco or Louisiana Hot Sauce, to taste

Sauté steak tips in a medium to large pot in the oil and garlic. Add parsley, onions, tomatoes, and beans. Continue stirring contents while adding the remaining ingredients. Reduce the heat to medium-low, and simmer the mixture until the meat is tender, about 30-40 minutes.

Serve with rice. Serves 2.

Positive Nutrition Exchanges: 3 fats & oils, 1 vegetable, 1 grain & baked good, 2 high-protein foods

Shish Kebab

This Armenian recipe is from Professor Lucy der Manuelian, who teaches at Tufts University, Medford, Massachusetts. She is a superb and enthusiastic cook.

1 lb. lamb, cut up
1 onion, finely chopped
1/4 teaspoon salt, to taste
1/8 teaspoon black pepper, to taste
1/2 teaspoon oregano, to taste
2 Tablespoons olive oil
2-3 tomatoes, cut in to wedges
1-1/2 large green pepper, cut into chunks

Combine lamb chunks with onion, salt, pepper, oregano, and olive oil. Marinate, covered and in the refrigerator, for 2-4 hours. Stir occasionally.

Alternate meat and vegetables on skewers, one skewer per person, and grill or broil, turning skewers until meat is well cooked.

Serves 3.

Positive Nutrition Exchanges: 3 fats & oils, 2 vegetables, 2 high-protein foods

Grilled "Cheater's Lamb"

Bob Hornstein says, "This is called Cheater's Lamb because the marinade is so simple to make: just open a bottle of your favorite French or Catalina salad dressing."

1 lb. lamb, any variety of cuts: chops, shank, riblets,
    butterfly leg of lamb, or even boneless lamb stew
    meat.
Salt and pepper, to taste
Bottle of French or Catalina style salad dressing
Fresh or dried rosemary, a few snips

Place lamb in glass dish in a single layer. Sprinkle with salt and pepper. Pour salad dressing over lamb, tossing to coat. Add a few snips of fresh or dried rosemary. Cover with plastic wrap, and refrigerate for 4 to 24 hours. Remove lamb from marinade, reserving liquid. Grill meat over medium flame, basting every few minutes and turning every few minutes so as not to burn the meat. Lamb is best when served medium well done, with just a tinge of pink left in the meat. Serves 2.

Positive Nutrition Exchanges: 2 fats & oils, 2 high-protein foods

Stuffed Cabbage, Russian Style

This hearty main course has many variations in Eastern Europe. This Russian version was given to Estelle Raiffa by her mother, who was born in Russia and emigrated to the United States when she was 15.

1 head green cabbage
1 lb. lean ground beef
1 cup white raisins, divided
1 egg, beaten
1 teaspoon salt
dash of pepper, to taste
1 large onion, minced
2 Tablespoons brown sugar
16 oz. tomato or V8 juice
1/4 teaspoon ground ginger, or 3 slices fresh ginger, or
    10 ginger snap cookies
sour cream (optional)

Remove and discard wilted outer leaves of the cabbage. Rinse and cut out some of the core of the cabbage to make it easier to remove the cabbage leaves. Place the cabbage in a large bowl and cover with boiling water. Let stand 1-2 minutes. Remove cabbage from water and carefully remove leaves that can be taken off easily. Repeat the process until you have all the large leaves you will need (about 8-9). The remainder of the cabbage can go into the casserole in a large chunk. Immerse the large leaves in cool water to cool them, then remove them to a dry plate.

Combine ground beef, 1/2 cup raisins, egg, salt, and pepper. Mix loosely, don't overhandle. Place about 3 or 4 tablespoons of the meat mixture on inner end of each cabbage leaf. Fold in sides of leaf and roll it up so that it is a tight bundle.

Combine the brown sugar, tomato juice, remaining 1/2 cup of

white raisins, and ginger to make the sauce. Arrange cabbage rolls over the minced onion in a heavy ungreased casserole. Pour sauce over all.

Cover and bake at 350° (for 2-3 hours). The longer the baking, the richer the gravy. Baste occasionally. If desired, serve with a dollop of sour cream on the plate, next to each cabbage roll.

Serves 4.

Positive Nutrition Exchanges: 1 fruit, 2 vegetables, 1 high-protein food

Tajine from Morocco

Dr. Amdiss, a Moroccan student in the Mason Fellows Program at Harvard University contributed this recipe.

1 medium onion, chopped
3 garlic cloves, chopped
2 Tablespoons butter
1 lb. ground beef
2 large fresh tomatoes, peeled and seeds removed
1 cup fresh parsley, chopped
3 teaspoons cumin powder
2 medium size potatoes, cooked and mashed
    (about 2 cups)
3 beaten eggs
2 teaspoons salt
pepper, to taste

Preheat oven to 350°. Sauté onion and garlic in butter over medium heat until golden in color. Combine the onion and garlic and remaining ingredients into the meat, and put into a buttered baking dish. Bake, uncovered, for 65 minutes. Remove from oven and let casserole stand for 10 minutes. Cut into squares and serve.
    Serves 3.

Positive Nutrition Exchanges: 2 fats & oils, 1 vegetable, 1 grain & baked good, 2 high-protein foods

Mexican Style Tamale Casserole

I found this recipe in the newsletter Bread and Circus
Markets and *tried it out and loved it. Bake it in a 8" x 11"
glass baking dish.—Estelle Raiffa*

1 lb. lean ground beef
1 cup tomato sauce
1 small onion, grated
1 clove garlic, chopped fine
1 egg
1 teaspoon cumin powder
1/4-1/2 teaspoon cayenne pepper (this is a very hot
    pepper), or use chili powder instead
1 Tablespoon chopped fresh cilantro
1 teaspoon salt, to taste
freshly ground black pepper, to taste

Preheat oven to 350°. In a bowl, mix all the ingredients and place in
buttered baking dish.

Topping:

2 cups coarse ground cornmeal
1/2 cup canned corn kernels
1/4 cup canola oil
1 1/2 cups buttermilk
2 Tablespoons sugar
1 teaspoon salt, to taste
black pepper, to taste
1/2 teaspoon baking powder
1 cup grated cheddar cheese

Mexican Style Tamale Casserole, continued

Combine cornmeal and corn in a bowl. Mix in remaining ingredients except cheese, combine well. Fold in cheese and spread topping over the meat mixture. Sprinkle some extra cheese over top. Bake for 40-50 minutes or until bubbling and brown. Do not overbake. Serve with plain yogurt on the side and salsa for garnish, if you like. Serves 3.

Positive Nutrition Exchanges: 1 dairy food, 3 fats & oils, 1 grain & baked good, 2 high-protein foods

Kalb's Goulash

This recipe was contributed by Rosemary Von Hopler Scully, who was born and raised in Vienna, Austria. She describes this recipe as "comfort food."

3 Tablespoons butter, divided
1 medium onion, chopped
1 lb. stewing veal
1 cup chicken broth
4-5 fresh mushrooms, sliced, or one small can of
     mushrooms, drained
1/2 teaspoon flour
1/3 cup heavy cream
1/4 cup brandy, optional

Sauté the onions in 2 tablespoons butter, over medium heat, until they are pale yellow. Add the pieces of veal, and brown the onions and veal together for about 5 minutes. Add chicken broth. Bring to a boil, and immediately reduce the heat to low. Cover the pot and simmer the meat for 1 1/2 to 2 hours.

Sauté the mushrooms in a separate pan with 1 tablespoon of butter until they are light brown. Add flour and mix it in with cooking mushrooms, or dissolve the flour in a little bit of cold water. Add the cooked mushrooms, heavy cream, and brandy to the meat.

Serve over noodles or rice. Serves 2.

Please note: If you use canned mushrooms, add the flour to a little bit of cold liquid before adding it to the meat.

Positive Nutrition Exchanges: 4 fats & oils, 1 vegetable, 2 high-protein foods

Chicken with Japanese-Style Sauce

Estelle Raiffa's daughter, Judith, suggested the ingredients for this particular sauce. The sautéed vegetables are added to enrich the flavor.

1 broiling chicken (2-3 lbs.) cut into quarters or eighths
1/3 cup soy sauce
1 teaspoon ground ginger
1 Tablespoon brown or white sugar
1 Tablespoon canola oil
1/4 teaspoon Tabasco sauce
juice of half a lemon, add 1/2 teaspoon grated lemon peel
    (optional)
1/2 cup orange juice, add 1/2 teaspoon grated orange peel
    (optional)
3-4 leeks, white and light green parts only. Wash carefully,
    splitting leeks down the center to get out any dirt. Cut
    leeks into large chunks.
2 Tablespoons canola oil
4-5 carrots, cleaned and cut into large chunks

Combine all ingredients except chicken, carrots vegetable oil, and carrots, and set aside. Preheat oven to 325°.

Wash and dry chicken pieces on paper towels, sprinkle with salt and pepper to taste. Place chicken pieces on a broiling pan and broil about 6 inches from heat. Turn pieces over when skin has browned and broil the other side the same way. When the skin has browned to your liking, remove the chicken to a glass baking dish. Pour the sauce over the chicken and place in the refrigerator for several hours to marinate.

Sauté leeks in oil in frying pan over medium heat. Add the carrots when the leeks are wilted and continue sautéeing for 2-3 minutes. Remove from heat.

Put sautéed vegetables in a baking dish. Place chicken pieces over the vegetables. Heat marinade and pour it over the chicken. Bake uncovered for 30 minutes.

Serves 3.

Positive Nutrition Exchanges: 3 fats & oils, 1 vegetable, 2 high-protein foods

Corned Beef and Cabbage, Irish Style

This recipe is from Maureen Maher Conneely who came from County Galway, to work for the Governor of Connecticut.

3-4 pounds corned beef (Try to buy the "first cut" which
    has less fat and more meat on it. The butcher can help
    you with this.)
1 small green cabbage, cut into quarters
1 large turnip, peeled and cut into chunks
4-5 large carrots, cleaned and cut into chunks (or use
    prepared carrots, about one half of a small bag)
2 medium potatoes, peeled and cut into chunks. You don't
    have to peel red potatoes.

Wash the beef with cold water. Place it in a deep pot, and cover with cold water. Bring water to a boil. Immediately reduce the heat to low, cover the pot and simmer for 2 1/2-3 hours. Test the meat with a fork to see if it is done. (Don't be surprised if the meat has shrunk, possibly by half.) Remove the meat from the pot and place in a covered dish with some of the cooking liquid to prevent the meat from drying out while the vegetables are cooking.

Add the cabbage, turnip, and carrots to the hot liquid, cover the pot and cook without the meat over medium heat for 25 minutes. Add potatoes and cook, covered, for another 10-15 minutes, until potatoes are tender.

To serve, slice the meat thinly, across the grain. (If the meat shreds, you are slicing it the wrong way.) Pour some of the cooking liquid over the meat. Serve the meat with mustard and a selection of the vegetables. *Note:* Save leftover sauce in the refrigerator and use for reheating any leftovers of the corned beef and vegetables. Serves 3.

**Positive Nutrition Exchanges: 2 vegetables, 1 grain & baked
    good, 2 high-protein foods**

Sauerkraut mit Wurstchen

This recipe was contributed by Renate Hafele of Germany. Surprisingly, the bacon fat doesn't make the dish taste greasy!

1/2 lb. (8 oz.) sauerkraut, package or can
4 frankfurters or 4 knockwurst (which I prefer), cut into
  bite-size pieces
8 strips of bacon, cut into one inch pieces
2-3 Tablespoons sour cream

Put sauerkraut, undrained, into sauce pan. Cover and cook on medium heat for 10 minutes. Add cut meat to the sauerkraut and cook over medium heat for 20 minutes. In a separate pan, fry bacon pieces. Pour the bacon and bacon fat onto the sauerkraut and meat after the latter has cooked for a total of 30 minutes. Add the sour cream to the sauerkraut and heat, but do not boil.

Serves 2.

Positive Nutrition Exchanges: 6 fats & oils, 1 vegetable, 1 high-protein food

Entrecôte Bordelaise

This recipe was contributed by Kathy Grenon of France.

1 medium onion, cut up small
2 Tablespoons butter
1/3 cup of red wine (Bordeaux type)
salt and pepper to taste
1 small steak (about 1/2 lb.), such as rib eye boneless, for
    one person

Cook onion in butter in frying pan over medium heat until it is pale yellow. Add the wine and bring to a boil. Add salt and pepper, to taste, and remove pan from heat. Broil the steak to your taste. Reheat the gravy quickly and pour over the steak.
    Serves 1

**Positive Nutrition Exchanges: 6 fats & oils, 2 high-protein
    foods**

There are a number of main course recipes that are really easy to prepare, and lend themselves to simple variations. The following recipes will serve one person; double the recipe to serve two.

Weiner Schnitzel (Viennese Veal)

While living in Vienna, we quickly came to appreciate the superb veal and poultry sold there.

6 oz. veal cutlet (a cutlet with the bone in is generally
    more tasty and tender than cutlets already boned)
Salt and pepper to taste
2 tablespoons flour for dusting
1 egg, beaten
1/4 cup plain bread crumbs
1 tablespoon butter, or light virgin olive oil or canola oil
1 slice of lemon, optional

If the cutlet has a bone, cut the bone away; you can use the bone in soup at a later time. Store bone in the freezer in a plastic bag. Place the veal between two sheets of wax paper, and pound the meat with a mallet until it is thin. Sprinkle the meat with salt and pepper, to taste. Dust the cutlet in flour, shake off excess. Dip the veal in the beaten egg and then in bread crumbs. Heat the butter or oil in a frying pan over medium heat; turn the heat down to low-medium and sauté the cutlet until it is light brown on each side (about 3-4 minutes per side). Serve with a slice of lemon, optional. This dish is good with baked or mashed potatoes or buttered noodles. Serves 1.

Positive Nutrition Exchanges: 3 fats & oils, 1 grain & baked good, 2 high-protein foods

Variation 1

When veal is turned over to cook the second side, put a piece of cheese on the cooked side, and it will soften by the time the second side is cooked. You can use Swiss, mozzarella, gruyere, or fontina cheese.

Weiner Schnitzel (Viennese Veal), continued
Variation 2

After veal is sautéed on both sides, set it aside on a plate, and cover loosely with aluminum foil. Quickly sauté 3 or 4 sliced mushrooms in the butter in the pan until they are light brown (2-3 minutes). Add 1/4 cup white wine or brandy to the mushrooms, and cook until half of the liquid remains. At this point, if you wish, you can also add 1-2 tablespoons of sour cream to the mushroom-wine gravy, and heat together (but don't boil). Pour the gravy over the veal and serve.

Variation 3 – Pariser Schnitzel

Pound the veal between two pieces of wax paper, until veal is thin. Sprinkle meat with salt and pepper, to taste. Dust the meat lightly in flour, and shake off excess. Heat butter or oil over medium heat until hot. Lower heat and sauté veal (3-4 minutes per side). Add a beaten egg to the veal in the pan, and cook until egg is thoroughly cooked on one side, then turn over the veal "omelet" and cook on the other side.

This is an extremely tasty way to serve veal, and can be found on the menu in Austrian restaurants.

Variation 4 – Veal Parmesan

Prepare the veal as you did for Weiner Schnitzel: meat is pounded, dust lightly in flour, dipped in beaten egg, then in bread crumbs, and lightly sautéed in butter or olive oil. Layer the veal with a prepared tomato sauce of your choice, for example a mushroom or primavera sauce. Sprinkle grated parmesan cheese (about 2-3 tablespoons) on top. If possible, use freshly grated cheese, since it has a better taste. Bake at 350° for 20 minutes. Serve with cooked pasta; you can use the extra sauce from the veal for the pasta.

Chicken Parmesan

*My nephew, Steven Schwartz gave me this excellent recipe.
Steve uses chicken breasts instead of veal. You can use chicken
breasts or chicken "tenders" in this recipe. Treat them the
same, except that the baking time is shorter for the "tenders."*

1 6-ounce chicken breast per person
Salt and pepper
Flour
1 egg, beaten
1/3 cup crushed onion and garlic croutons
2 tablespoons butter or light virgin olive oil
1/2 cup white wine, divided
1 slice mozzarella cheese

Wash and dry chicken breast and sprinkle with salt and pepper.
Dip chicken breast (or chicken tenders) lightly in flour and shake
off excess. Dip chicken in beaten egg and roll in crouton crumbs.
Sauté chicken in heated butter or olive oil over low-medium heat
until chicken is lightly browned (about 3-4 minutes per side). Add
1/4 cup of wine to the frying pan and cover the pan so that chicken
steams for 1-2 minutes in the wine. Turn the chicken over and add
remaining 1/4 cup of wine, cover and steam the chicken on the
second side for another 1-2 minutes.

Layer the chicken breasts and sauce in a buttered baking dish.
Top with cheese. Bake the chicken, uncovered, at 350° for 30 min-
utes. (If using chicken tenders, baking time will be 20 minutes.)
Serves 1.

**Positive Nutrition Exchanges: 6 fats & oils, 2 high-protein
  foods**

Chili con Carne

Barbara Miranda, a legislative assistant to a state representative, likes to serve this dish at parties and political gatherings.

1 lb. lean ground beef
14-16-oz. can red kidney beans, undrained
14-16-oz. can whole tomatoes, undrained
1 large package dry chili seasoning mix (I recommend
    Durkee's)
1-2 teaspoons chili powder, optional, to taste
1/2 cup grated cheddar cheese
1/2 cup sour cream
1/2 cup red onions
Tortilla chips

Brown the ground beef in a frying pan, and drain off fat. Transfer the sautéed beef to a large pot. Add kidney beans, tomatoes, chili seasoning, and chili powder. Bring the mixture to a boil. Turn heat to low and simmer, stirring occasionally, for 15 minutes.

Put the grated cheese, sour cream, and red onions into 3 separate small bowls. Serve the chili in a soup bowl. Add cheese, sour cream, and onions over the top of the chili, as desired. Serve with a basket of tortilla chips.

Serves 4.

**Positive Nutrition Exchanges: 2 fats & oils, 1 vegetable,
  2 high-protein foods**

Chicken Paprikash

This recipe was contributed by Maria Rabar, of Hungary (from the IIASA cookbook). It's one of the simplest, yet most delicious dishes in this book.

3 tablespoons canola oil
3 lbs. cut up chicken
2 large onions, cut up
1 heaping teaspoon sweet Hungarian paprika
2 cups sour cream (do not use non-fat sour cream)

Wash and dry chicken with paper towels, and salt to taste Heat the oil over medium-high heat in a heavy pan or pot. Add the chicken pieces, and sear the chicken over medium-high heat for about 6-7 minutes. Remove the chicken to a plate, and set aside.

Brown the onions in the remaining oil in the pot. When the onions are pale yellow, about 3-4 minutes, sprinkle the paprika over the onions and mix together. Add the chicken to the onion/paprika and mix together. Lower the heat to low-simmer, cover the pot, and simmer for about 50 minutes. Stir once or twice during the cooking.

You may be surprised to see about a cup of gravy has been made. After the chicken has simmered for 50 minutes, add the sour cream to the pot, stirring it into the gravy. Cover the pot and simmer over low heat for 10 minutes. Serve the chicken and gravy with flat cooked noodles.

Serves 4.

Positive Nutrition Exchanges: 4 fats & oils, 2 high-protein foods

references

The following is a list of references that were consulted during the writing of this book.

Obviously the list is lengthy and will be of greatest value to health care professional readers who wish to amplify their clinical knowledge. Lay readers should not be put off entirely, however, because many of the articles are highly accessible.

In any event, we have attached an asterisk (*) to the references we feel are most important.

*Abrams B, Duncan D, Hertz-Picciotta I: A prospective study of dietary intake and acquired immune deficiency syndrome in HIV-seropositive homosexual men. *Journal of AIDS* 1993; 6:949-958.

Anderson RM, May RA: Understanding the AIDS pandemic. *Scientific American* 1992; 390:58-66.

Anonymous: Malnutrition and weight loss in patients with AIDS. *Nutrition Reviews* 1989; 47:354-356.

Anonymous: What do we know about the mechanism of weight loss in AIDS? *Nutrition Reviews* 1990; 48:153-155.

Bandy CE, Guyer LK, Perkin JE, Probart CK, Rodrick GE: Nutrition attitudes and practices of individuals who are infected with human immunodeficiency virus and who live in south Florida. *Journal of the American Dietetic Association* 1993; 93:70-72.

*Baum MK, Shor-Posner G, Lu Y, et al: Micronutrients and HIV-1 disease progression. *AIDS* 1995; 9:1051-1056.

*Beal JF, Olson R, Laubenstein L, Morales JO, Bellman P, Yangco B, Lefkowitz L, Plasse TF, Shepard KV: Dronabinol as a treatment for anorexia associated with weight loss in patients with AIDS. *Journal of Pain and Symptom Management* 1995; 10:89-97.

Begin ME, Manki MS, Horrobin DF: Plasma fatty acid levels in patients with acquired immune deficiency syndrome and in controls. *Prostaglandins, Leukotrienes, and Essential Fatty Acids* 1989; 37:135-137.

*Bell SJ, Mascioli EA, Bistrian BR, Babayan VK, Blackburn GL: Alternative lipid sources for enteral and parenteral nutrition: long- and medium-chain triglycerides, structured triglycerides, and fish oil. *Journal of the American Dietetic Association* 1991; 91:74-78.

*Bell SJ, Mascioli EA, Forse RA, Bistrian BR: Nutrition support of the patient with the human immunodeficiency virus. *Parasitology* 1993; 107:1-15.

*Bell SJ, Chavali S, Forse RA: Cytokine influence on the human immunodeficiency virus (HIV): action, prevalence, and treatment. IN: Forse RA, Bell SJ, Kabbash LG (eds.). *Diet, Nutrition, and Immunity.* CRC Press: Boca Raton, FL, 1994, chapter 9.

*Bell SJ, Chavali S, Bistrian BR, Connolly CA, Utsunomiya T, Forse RA: Dietary fish oil and cytokines and eicosanoid production during human immunodeficiency virus infection. *Journal of Parenteral and Enteral Nutrition* 1996:20:43-49

Birx, DL, Redfield RR, Tencer K, Fowler A, Burke DS, Tosato G: Induction of Interleukin-6 during human immunodeficiency virus infection. *Blood* 1990; 76:2303-2310.

Blackburn GL, Bistrian BR, Maini BS, Schlamm HT, Smith MF: Nutritional and metabolic assessment of the hospitalized patient. *Journal of Parenteral and Enteral Nutrition* 1977; 1:11-22.

*Blackburn GL, Bell SJ: Eutrophia in patients with HIV infection and early AIDS with novel nutrient "cocktail": is this the first food for special medical purpose? *Nutrition* 1993; 9:554-556.

Bogden JD, Baker H, Frank O, Perez G, Kemp F, Bruening K, Louria D: Micronutrient status and human immunodeficiency virus (HIV) infection. *New York Academy of Science* 1990; 587:189-195.

references

*Byrne TA, Morrissey TB, Nattakom TV, Ziegler TR, Wilmore DW. Growth hormone, glutamine, and a modified diet enhance nutrient absorption in patients with severe short bowel syndrome. *Journal of Parenteral and Enteral Nutrition* 1995; 19:296-302.

*Chlebowski RT, Grosvenor MB, Bernhard NH, Morales LS, Bulcavage LM: Nutritional status, gastrointestinal dysfunction, and survival in patients with AIDS. *American Journal of Gastroenterology* 1989; 84:1288-1293.

*Chlebowski RT, Beall G, Grosvenor M, Lillington L, Weintraub N, Ambler C, Richards EW, Abbruzzese BC, McCamish MA, Cope FO: Long-term effects of early nutritional support with new enterotropic peptide-based formula vs. standard enteral formula in HIV-infected patients: randomized prospective trial. *Nutrition* 1993; 9:507-512.

Dinarello CA, Endres S, Meydani SN, Meydani M, Hellerstein MK: Interleukin-1, anorexia, and dietary fatty acids. *New York Academy of Science* 1990; 587:332-338.

*Dworkin BM, Rosenthal WS, Wormser GP, Weiss L: Selenium deficiency in the acquired immunodeficiency syndrome. *Journal of Parenteral and Enteral Nutrition* 1986; 10:405-407.

*Dworkin BM, Wormser GP, Axelrod F, Pierre N, Schwarz E, Schwartz E, Seaton T: Dietary intake in patients with acquired immunodeficiency syndrome (AIDS), patients with AIDS-related complex, and serologically positive human immunodeficiency virus patients: correlations with nutritional status. *Journal of Parenteral and Enteral Nutrition* 1990; 14:605-609.

*Dwyer JT, Bye RL, Holt PL, Lauze SR: Unproven nutrition therapies for AIDS: what is the evidence? *Nutrition Today* 1988; Mar/Apr: 25-33.

Dwyer JT: Nutrition support of HIV+ patients *Henry Ford Hospital Medical Journal* 1991; 39:60-65.

Endres S, Ghorbani R, Kelley VE, Georgilis K, Lonnemann G, van der Meer JWM, Cannon JG, Rogers TS, Klimpner MS, Weber PC, Schaeffer EJ, Wolff SM, Dinarello CA: The effect of dietary supplementation with n-3 polyunsaturated fatty acids on the synthesis of interleukin-1 and tumor necrosis factor by mononuclear cells. *New England Journal of Medicine* 1989; 320:265-271.

Erickson KL: Dietary fat modulation of immune response. *Int J Immunopharmacology* 1986; 8:529-543.

Feingold KR, Serio MK, Adi S, Moser AH, Grunfeld C: Tumor necrosis factor-stimulated hepatic lipid synthesis and secretion. *Endocrinology* 1989; 124:2336-2342.

Feingold KR, Soued M, Serio MK, Moser AH, Dinarello CA, Grunfeld C: Multiple cytokines stimulate hepatic lipid synthesis in vivo. *Endocrinology* 1989; 125:267-274.

*Feingold KR, Adi S, Staprans I, Moser AH, Neese R, Verdier JA, Doerrler W, Grunfeld C: Diet affects the mechanisms by which TNF stimulates hepatic triglyceride production. *American Journal of Physiology* 1990; 259:E177-E184.

Fields-Gardner C: A review of mechanisms of wasting in HIV disease. *Nutrition in Clinical Practice* 1995; 10:167-175.

Fong Y, Lowry SF: Cytokines and the cellular response to injury and infection. In: Wilmore DL, Brennan MF, Harken AH, Holcroft JW, Meakins JL (eds). Trauma IV. *Scientific American,* 1990, chapter 7.

Gorbach SL, Knox TA, Roubenoff R: Interactions between nutrition and infection with human immunodeficiency virus. *Nutrition Reviews* 1993; 51:226-234.

*Grunfeld C, Wilking H, Neese R, Gavin LA, Moser AH, Gulli R, Serio MK, Feingold KR: Persistence of the hypertriglyceridemic effect of tumor necrosis factor despite development of tachyphylaxis to its anorectic/cachetic effects in rats. *Cancer Research* 1989; 49:2554-2560.

*Grunfeld C, Pang M, Shimizu L, Shigenaga JK, Jensen P, Feingold KR: Preservation of short-term energy balance in clinically stable patients with AIDS. *American Journal of Clinical Nutrition* 1990; 51:7-13.

Grunfeld C, Kotler DP, Shigenaga JK, Doerrler W, Tierney A, Wang J, Person RN, Feingold KR: Circulating interferon-a levels and hypertriglyceridemia in the acquired immunodeficiency syndrome. *American Journal of Medicine* 1991; 90:154-162.

*Grunfeld C, Pang M, Shimizu L, Shigenaga JK, Jensen P, Feingold KR: Resting energy expenditure, caloric intake, and short-term weight change in human immunodeficiency virus infection and the acquired immunodeficiency syndrome. *American Journal of Clinical Nutrition* 1992; 55:455-460.

*Grunfeld C, Feingold KR: Metabolic disturbances and wasting in the acquired immunodeficiency syndrome. *New England Journal of Medicine* 1992; 327:329-337.

Grunfeld C, Feingold KR: Tumor necrosis factor, interleukin, and interferon induced changes in lipid metabolism as part of host defense. *Proceedings of the Society of Experimental Biology and Medicine* 1992; 200:224-227.

Guenter PA, Muurahainen N, Cohan CR, Turner JL: Relationships among nutritional status, disease progression, and survival in HIV infection. *Journal of AIDS* 1993; 6:1130-1138.

Harakeh S, Neidzwiecki A, Jariwalla RJ; Mechanistic aspects of ascorbate inhibition of human immunodeficiency virus. *Chemico-Biologico* 1994; 91:207-215.

references

*Hellerstein MK, Meydani SN, Meydani M, Wu K, Dinarello CA: Interleukin-1-induced anorexia in the rat. *Journal of Clinical Investigation* 1989; 84:228-235.

Hellerstein MK, Kahn J, Mudie H, Viteri F: Current approach to the treatment of human immunodeficiency virus-associated weight loss: pathophysiologic consideration and emerging management strategies. *Seminars in Oncology* 1990; 17:17-33.

*Hellerstein MK, Grunfeld C, Wu K, Christiansen M, Kaemper S, Kletke C, Shackleton CHL: Increased de novo hepatic lipogenesis in human immunodeficiency virus infection. *Journal of Clinical Endocrinology Metabolism* 1993; 76:559-565.

Henry K: Alternative therapies for AIDS. *Minnesota Medicine* 1988; 71:297-299.

*Ho WZ, Douglas SD: Glutathione and N-acetylcysteine suppression of immunodeficiency virus replication in human monocyte/macrophage in vitro. *AIDS Research and Human Retrovirus* 1992; 8:1249-1253.

*Hommes MJT, Romijin JA, Endert E, Sauerwein HP: Resting energy expenditure and substrate oxidation in human immunodeficiency virus (HIV-1)-infected asymptomatic men: HIV affects host metabolism in the early asymptomatic stage. *American Journal of Clinical Nutrition* 1991; 54:311-315.

Hommes MJT, Romijin JA, Endert E, Schattenkerk JKM, Sauerwein HP: Basal fuel homeoastasis in symptomatic human immunodeficiency virus infection. *Clinical Science* 1991; 80:359-365.

Janson DD, Teasley KM: Parenteral nutrition in the management of gastrointestinal Kaposi's sarcoma in a patient with AIDS. *American Society of Hospital Pharmacy* 1988; 7:536-544.

Jones PD, Shelley L, Wakefield D: Tumor necrosis factor-a in advanced HIV infection in the absence of AIDS-related secondary infections. *Journal of AIDS* 1992; 5:1266-1271.

Keusch GT, Thea DM: Malnutrition in AIDS. *Medical Clinics of North America* 1993; 77:795-814.

Kotler DP, Wang J, Pierson RN: Body composition studies in patients with acquired immunodeficiency syndrome. *American Journal of Clinical Nutrition* 1985; 42:1255-1265.

*Kotler DP, Tierney AR, Wang J, Pierson RN: Magnitude of body-cell-mass depletion and the timing of death from wasting in AIDS. *American Journal of Clinical Nutrition* 1989; 50:444-447.

Kotler DP, Tierney AR, Brenner SK, Couture S, Wang J, Pierson RN: Preservation of short-term energy balance in clinically stable patients with AIDS. *American Journal of Clinical Nutrition* 1990; 51:7-13.

*Kotler DP, Tierney AR, Culpepper-Morgan JA, Wang J, Pierson RN: Effect of home total parenteral nutrition on body composition in patients with acquired immunodeficiency syndrome. *Journal of Parenteral and Enteral Nutrition* 1990; 14:454-458.

Kotler DP: Biological and clinical features of HIV infection. IN: *Gastrointestinal and Nutritional Manifestations of the Acquired Immunodeficiency Syndrome,* Kotler DP (ed). Raven Press, New York, 1991, pp. 1-16.

*Kotler, Tierney AR, Ferraro R, Cuff P, Wang J, Pierson RN, Heymsfield SB: Enteral alimentation and repletion of body cell mass in malnourished patients with AIDS. *American Journal of Clinical Nutrition* 1991; 53:149-154.

Lacey JM, Wilmore DW: Is glutamine a conditionally essential amino acid? *Nutrition Reviews* 1990; 48:297-306.

*Lahdevireta K. Maury CPJ, Teppo AM, Repo H: Elevated levels of circulating cachectin/tumor necrosis factor in patients with acquired immunodeficiency syndrome. *American Journal of Medicine* 1988; 85:289-291.

Lau AS, Livesey JF: Endotoxin induction of tumor necrosis factor is enhanced by acid-labile interferon-a in acquired immunodeficiency syndrome. *Journal of Clinical Investigation* 1989; 84:738-743.

Lau AS, Der SD, Read SE, Williams BRG: Regulation of tumor necrosis factor receptor expression by acid-labile interferon-a from AIDS sera. *AIDS Research and Human Retrovirus* 1991; 7:545-552.

*Macallan DC, Noble C, Baldwin C, et al: Energy expenditure and wasting in human immunodeficiency virus infection. *New England Journal of Medicine* 1995; 333:83-88.

*Macallan DC, Noble C, Baldwin C, Foskett M, McManus T, Griffin GE: Prospective analysis of patterns of weight change in stage IV human immunodeficiency virus infection. *American Journal of Clinical Nutrition* 1993; 58:417-424.

*Melchior JC, Salmon D, Riguad D, Leport C, Bouvet E, Detruchis P, Vilde JL, Vachon F, Coulaud JP, Apfelbaum M: Resting energy expenditure is increased in stable, malnourished HIV-infected patients. *American Journal of Clinical Nutrition* 1991; 53:437-441.

Melchior JAC, Raguin G, Boulier A, Bouvet E, Riguad D, Matheron S, Casalino E, Vilde JL, Vachon F, Coulaud JP, Apfelbaum M: Resting energy expenditure in human immunodeficiency virus-infected patients: comparison between patients with and without secondary infections. *American Journal of Clinical Nutrition* 1993; 57:614-619.

Meydani SN: Dietary modulation of cytokine production and biologic functions. *Nutrition Reviews* 1990; 48:361-369.

references

Meydani SN, Barklund MP, Liu S, Meydani M, Miller RA, Cannon JF, Morrow FD, Rocklin R, Bulumberg JB: Vitamin E supplementation enhances cell-mediated immunity in healthy elderly subjects. *American Journal of Clinical Nutrition* 1990; 52:557-563.

Molina JM, Scadden DT, Byrm R, Dinarello CA, Groopman JE: Production of tumor necrosis factor-a and interleukin-1 by monocytic cells infected with human immunodeficiency virus. *Journal of Clinical Investigation* 1989; 84:733-737.

Mukau L, Talamini MA, Sitzmann JV, Burns C, McGuire ME: Long-term central venous access vs. other home therapies: complications in patients with acquired immunodeficiency syndrome. *Journal of Parenteral and Enteral Nutrition* 1992; 16:455-459.

Munis JR, Richman DD, Kornbluth RS: Human immunodeficiency virus-1 infection of macrophages in vitro neither induces tumor necrosis factor (TNF)/cachectin gene expression nor alters TNF/cachectin induction lipopolysaccharide. *Journal of Clinical Investigation* 1990; 85:591-596.

Norwalk MA, McMichael AJ: How HIV defeats the immune system. *Scientific American* 1995; 273:58-65.

Olmsted L, Schrauzer GN, Flores-Arce M, Dowd J: Selenium supplementation of symptomatic human immunodeficiency virus infected patients. *Biological Trace Element Research* 1989; 20:59-65.

O'Sullivan P, Linke RA, Dalton S: Evaluation of body weight and nutritional status among AIDS patients. *Journal of the American Dietetic Association* 1985; 85:1483-1484.

*Ott M, Lembcke B, Fisher H, Jager R, Polat H, Geier H, Rech M, Staszeswki S, Helm EB, Caspary WF: Early changes of body composition in human immunodeficiency virus-infected patients: tetrapolar body impedance analysis indicates significant malnutrition. *American Journal of Clinical Nutrition* 1993; 57:15-19.

Pantaleo G, Grazio C, Fauci AS: The immunogenesis of human immunodeficiency infection. *New England Journal of Medicine* 1993; 328:327-335.

Pantaleo G, Grazios C, Demarest JF, Butini L, Montroni M, Fox CH, Orenstein JM, Kotler DP, Fauci AS: HIV infection is active and progressive in lymphoid tissue during clinically latent stage of disease. *Nature* 1993; 362:355-358.

Patton JS, Peters PM, McCabe J, Crase D, Hansen S, Chen AB, Liggitt D: Development of partial tolerance to the gastrointestinal effects of high doses of recombinant tumor necrosis factor-a in rodents. *Journal of Clinical Investigation* 1987; 80:1587-1596.

Phair JP. Estimating prognosis in HIV-1 infection. *Annals of Internal Medicine* 1993; 118:742-743.

Poli G, Fauci AS: The effect of cytokines and pharmacologic agents on chronic HIV infection. *AIDS Research and Human Retrovirus* 1992; 8:191-197.

Poli G. Fauci AS: Cytokine modulation of HIV expression. *Seminars in Immunology* 1993; 5:165-173.

Pomposelli JJ, Mascioli EA, Bistrian BR, Lopes SM, Blackburn GL: Attenuation of the febrile response in guinea pigs by fish oil enriched diets. *Journal of Parenteral and Enteral Nutrition* 1989; 13:136-140.

Raiten DJ: Nutrition and HIV infection: a review and evaluation of the extant knowledge of the relationship between nutrition and HIV infection. Bethesda: Life Sciences Research Office, Federation of American Societies for Experimental Biology. *Nutrition in Clinical Practice* 1991; 6:1-94.

Rakower D, Galvin TA: Nourishing the HIV-infected adult. *Holistic Nutrition Practice* 1989; 3:26-37.

Raviglione MC, Battan R, Pablos-Mendez A, Aceves-Casilla P, Mullen MP, Taranta A: Infection association with Hickman catheters in patients with acquired immunodeficiency syndrome. *American Journal of Medicine* 1989; 86:780-786.

Recommended Dietary Allowances. 10th edition, National Research Council. National Academy Press, 1989.

Reddy MM, Sorrell SJ, Lange M, Grieco MH: Tumor necrosis factor and HIV P24 antigen levels in serum of HIV-infected populations. *Journal of AIDS* 1988; 1:436-440.

Redfield RR: The Walter Reed Staging classification for HTLV-III/LAV infection. *New England Journal of Medicine* 1986; 314:131-132.

Redfield RR, Burke DS: HIV infection: the clinical picture. *Scientific American* 1988; 259:90-100.

Resler SS: Nutrition care of AIDS patients. *Journal of the American Dietetic Association* 1988; 88:828-832.

Roederer M, Staal FJT, Raju PA, Ela SW, Herzenberg LA, Herzenberg LA: Cytokine-stimulated human immunodeficiency virus replication is inhibited by N-acetyl-L-cysteine. *Proceedings of the National Academy of Science (USA)* 1990; 87:4884-4888.

*Roederer M, Ela SW, Staal FJT, Herzenberg LA, Herzenberg LA: N-acetyl-cysteine: a new approach to anti-HIV therapy. *AIDS Research and Human Retrovirus* 1992; 8:209-215.

Rombeau JL, Caldwell MD: *Clinical Nutrition: Enteral and Tube Feeding.* 2nd Edition. Philadelphia: W.B. Saunders, 1990.

Ruegg CL, Engelman EG: Impaired immunity in AIDS. *Annals of the New York Academy of Science* 1990; 616:307-317.

Schwartz JH, Bistrian BR: The role of cytokines in intermediary metabolism. In: *Cellular and Molecular Aspects of Endotoxin Reactions.* Eds: Nowotny A, Spitzer JJ, Ziegler EJ. Amsterdam: Elsevier, 1990; pp. 427-445.

Schwenk A, Burger B, Wessel D, Stutzer H, Ziegenhagen D, Diehl V, Schrappe M: Clinical risk factors for malnutrition in HIV-1 infected patients. *AIDS* 1993; 7:1213-1219.

Scott-Algara D, Vuillier F, Marasescu M, de Saint Martin J, Gighiero G: Serum levels of IL-2, IL-1a, TNF-a, and soluble receptor of IL-2 in HIV-1-infected patients. *AIDS Research and Human Retrovirus* 1991; 7:381-386.

Shabert J, Ehrlich N: *The Ultimate Nutrient Glutamine.* Avery Publishing Group, Garden City Park, NJ, 1994.

*Singer P, Rothkopf MM, Kvetan V, Kirvela O, Gaare J, Askanazi J: Risks and benefits of home parenteral nutrition in the acquired immunodeficiency syndrome. *Journal of Parenteral and Enteral Nutrition* 1991; 15:75-79.

Singer P, Rubinstein A, Askanazi J, Calvelli T, Lazarus T, Kirvela O, Katz DP: clinical and immunologic effects of lipid-based parenteral nutrition in AIDS. *Journal of Parenteral and Enteral Nutrition* 1992; 16:165-167.

Singer P, Katz DP, Dillon L, Kirvela O, Lazarus T, Askanazi J: Nutritional aspects of the acquired immunodeficiency syndrome. *American Journal of Gastroenterology* 1992; 87:265-273.

*Staal FJT, Roederer M, Raju FA, Anderson MT, Ela SW, Herzenberg LA, Herzenberg LA: Antioxidants inhibit stimulation of HIV transcription. *AIDS Research and Human Retrovirus* 1993; 9:299-306.

*Stack JA, Bell SJ, Burke PA, Forse RA: Use of oral supplements in patients with human immunodeficiency virus infection. *Journal of the American Dietetic Association* 1996; 96:337-341.

Stein TP, Nutinsky C, Condolluci D, Schluter MD, Leskiw MJ: Protein and energy substrate metabolism in AIDS patients. *Metabolism* 1990; 39:876-881.

Stevenson M, Bukrinsky M, Haggerty: HIV-1 replication and potential targets for intervention. *AIDS Research and Human Retrovirus* 1992; 8:107-117.

Tang AM, Graham H, Kirby AJ, McCall LD, Willet WC, Saah AJ: Dietary micronutrient intake and risk of progression to acquired immunodeficiency syndrome (AIDS) in human immunodeficiency virus type 1 (HIV-1)-infected homosexual men. *American Journal of Epidemiology* 1993; 138:937-951.

Task Force on Nutrition Support in AIDS. Guidelines for nutrition support in AIDS. *Nutrition* 1989; 5:39-46.

Tchekmedyian NS: Treatment of anorexia with megestrol acetate. *Nutrition in Clinical Practice* 1993; 8:115-118.

*Trujillo EB, Borlase BC, Bell SJ, Guenther KJ, Swails W, Queen PM, Trujillo JR: Assessment of nutritional status nutrient intake, and nutrition support in AIDS patients. *Journal of the American Dietetic Association* 1992; 92:477-478.

*Tuttle-Newhall JE, Veerabagu MP, Mascioli E, Blackburn GL: Nutrition and metabolic management of AIDS during acute illness. *Nutrition* 1993; 9:240-244.

VonRoenn JH, Armstrong D, Kotler DP, Cohn DL, Klimas NG, Tchelcmedyian NS, Cone L, Brennan PJ, Weitzman SA: Megestrol acetate in patients with AIDS-related cachexia. *Annals of Internal Medicine* 1994; 121:393-399.

Von Sydow M, Sonnerborg A, Gaines H, Strannegard O: Interferon-alpha and tumor necrosis factor-alpha in serum of patients in various stages of HIV-1 infection. *AIDS Research and Human Retrovirus* 1991; 7:375-380.

Waites L, Mello L: Long-term parenteral nutrition support in a 30-year-old man. *AIDS Patient Care* 1991; June:60-61.

Weiss L, Haeffner-Cavaillon N, Laude M, Gilquin J, Kazatchkine MD: HIV infection is associated with the spontaneous production of interleukin-1 (IL-1) in vivo and with an abnormal release of IL-1a in vitro. *AIDS* 1989; 3:695-699.

Yarchoan R, Mitsuya H, Broder S: The immunology of HIV infection: implications for therapy. *AIDS Research and Human Retrovirus* 1992; 8:1023-1031.

*Young LC, Gatzen C, Wilmore K, Wilmore DW: Glutamine (Gln) supplementation fails to increase plasma Gln levels in asymptomatic HIV+ individuals. *Journal of the American Dietetic Association (supp)* 1992; abstract 88.

*Ziegler TR, Young LS, Benfell K, Byrne TA, Wilmore DW: Clinical and metabolic efficacy of glutamine-supplemented parenteral nutrition after bone marrow transplantation. *Annals of Internal Medicine* 1992; 116:821-828.

Index